OLDERS' VOICES

WISDOM GLADLY SHARED BY THE
CHRONOLOGICALLY GIFTED

JANET BENNER, PH.D.

Copyright © 2023 Janet Benner, PH.D.
All rights reserved
First Edition

NEWMAN SPRINGS PUBLISHING
320 Broad Street
Red Bank, NJ 07701

First originally published by Newman Springs Publishing 2023

ISBN 979-8-88763-626-9 (Paperback)
ISBN 979-8-88763-627-6 (Digital)

Printed in the United States of America

Dedicated to the Memory of
Ella Mae Brown Ramsey
1932–2022

INTRODUCTION

At every medical appointment, one is asked, "What is your date of birth?" That has become your second name. For me, it's 12-9-36. To ensure anonymity, the contributors to this are known only as their birth dates. So while this whole affair will not be about me, it will be from my perspective, how things look to me from this angle—my 86-year-old angle.

I remember when I had my first baby, my thought was no one really told me what this child birthing was all about. I didn't know this or that or the other thing. That's the way I feel about aging. No one told us it would be like this.

I've interviewed and gotten the stories of many of my 70- and 80-something neighbors and friends (including one 68-year-old and one 99-year-old). Initially, I was calling the book *Eighty Something*, then decided people in their 70s could add much. The title changed to *Olders' Voices*.

I live in a neighborhood where several older people live. Some of them have participated. I've told my own story and asked other people from all over the United States who are olders to participate. It's been interesting who will write their story and who will not. All but one or two took months with prodding to get it done. I think it was all a part of the older story. Things just take us longer to get done. And I also surmised that just as when we're 20 or 50, everyone has their own style and way of being and doing.

One of the biggest things about this oldness is the isolation. I am hoping that the middle-aged children of Olders will read this and understand how wonderful it is for Mama and Daddy Olders to receive a regular phone call or visit from their offspring.

So here I am with the others, writing about what this is all like. For me, like so many, the pandemic was a setback. I did not see people or talk to people much for two years. One of my main activities was talking to and helping my friend Ellie, who was also my daughter's mother-in-law. She passed away a few months ago at age 89.

This was a horrible loss for me. If I was making potato salad, I always made sure I made some for Ellie too. Same with pasta sauce. I called her or went by to see her every day at about four in the afternoon, that time of day when everything I had planned for the day was done and it was not yet time to make dinner. We talked about all this getting-old stuff, and we gossiped about our children and how they don't always do what we think they should.

She became more and more infirm with trips in and out of hospitals. Her great conviction was that doctors and others were trying to fix her, and she could no longer be fixed. Just let her go.

And go she did. We visited her at five thirty at the hospice where she had just been deposited that afternoon. Lovely. It was a lovely place with lovely people. A good place to die. So we visited her that afternoon, and she died at seven o'clock that evening. I was so happy that we had stopped to see her before she left. I would have felt bad about it the rest of my life had we not. Her being gone left what felt like a big hole in my life. This book, as you probably have seen, is dedicated to Ellie. That's one thing about getting old, the loss. We lose people every day, and there's nothing we can do about it.

As I prepared to do this book, I thought about what I would ask the Olders about their own getting old experience. Following is the list of questions I suggested they address in narrative form as their contribution to this book. I wanted it to be in their own voices. I now wish I had asked if they still drive and about music and a little something about their knowledge of technology. Some answered those questions anyway.

QUESTIONS FOR OLDERS

BIRTH DATE?

1. HOW DO YOU *FEEL*?
   A. EMOTIONALLY?
   B. PHYSICALLY?
   C. ABOUT YOURSELF?

2. WHAT IS YOUR PHYSICAL CONDITION? PLEASE DESCRIBE.

3. ARE YOU STILL SEXUALLY ACTIVE—FREQUENTLY, OCCASIONALLY, NEVER?

4. DO YOU USE A CANE? A WALKER? WHAT'S THAT LIKE FOR YOU?

5. HAVE YOU FAMILY? WHAT? CHILDREN, HOW MANY, GRANDCHILDREN, HOW MANY? DO YOU LIVE ALONE OR WITH WHOM?

6. BEFORE BECOMING AN OLDER, WHAT DID YOU DO? HOW DO YOU FEEL ABOUT THAT NOW?
   A. WAS IT WORTHWHILE?
   B. DO YOU MISS WORKING?
   C. WERE YOU GOOD AT WHAT YOU DID?
   D. DID YOU MAKE ENOUGH MONEY?

7. AND NOW, ARE FINANCIAL CONSIDERATIONS AN ISSUE? OR DO YOU HAVE ENOUGH AND WHAT YOU NEED?

8. DO YOU HAVE A RELIGION? SPIRITUALITY? DO YOU BELIEVE IN LIFE AFTER DEATH?

WHAT ELSE SHOULD WE KNOW ABOUT YOU FOR THE BOOK WE'RE ALL GOING TO WRITE? YOU WILL BE IDENTIFIED ONLY BY YOUR BIRTH DATE.

THANK YOU SO MUCH FOR PARTICIPATING IN THIS EFFORT.

1

8-17-50

Ah, growing older—A Tale of Two Bodies. It was the best of times. It was the worst of times. Olders seem to have two types of days, painful and somewhat pain-free. The trouble is you don't know which day you're going to have until it arrives. This is problematic for planning purposes, but does make for some interesting or humorous choices when you have to improvise and go to Plan B. Some days you feel downright victorious when the only thing you've accomplished is taking a shower. It's a crapshoot.

Emotionally, it's tricky. Things seem to change rather rapidly as you age. Life goes along for years, you work, find your tribe, and make lifelong friends. Except now the health of your friends is failing and this changes those plans. Some move away to be closer to their families, some move to warmer climates, some move to nursing homes and some die. It's heartbreaking to lose anyone, but particularly a close friend, someone you've known since childhood. It's especially cruel to lose them to dementia or Alzheimer's. First you lose your history with them, the connection that made them and your relationship so special. You can no longer call to tell them something that only they would understand. Be it slow or fast, watching their decline is painful. Finally, they lose their battle. Losing a friend is hard. Losing him or her twice is harder.

No one tells Olders that the body may be looking a bit worn, but you still feel young inside. I think we should be told; it gives us hope. It makes us feel we can handle the challenges of living older and we can live well. We may not be able to accomplish all the physical feats we easily achieved in our youth, but we have those memories. Sometimes that's all that's needed to get us through any specific situation. One of the things I do is find clever little cartoons and pictures in FB and other places and I send them to a list of friends. (It's the only superpower I have—wink, wink—not a huge thing, but may brighten the day for someone.)

Given my age and family medical history, my health is good. Although my inherited spinal problems and arthritis are a bitch, I can still get around and am luckier than many others my age. Mobility is a big issue and I have a better understanding now of those who have this challenge. As most things in life, if you haven't experienced it, you have no idea what it's like. Now I get what my father once said to me, "It's scary when your body starts to betray you."

Regarding sexual activity, the frequency and the days of marathon gymnastic exploits are long gone, they are replaced with the intimacy that originates from maturity and decades of life experiences with your partner. However, daily hugs and kisses are a must. Also, do not underestimate the power of holding hands, laughing and dancing around the kitchen.

I use neither a cane nor a walker yet, but I'm pretty sure that's likely in my future. For now, holding on to the shopping cart seems to be working for me when I have to be in a store for a long time. Perhaps I'll be one of those who decorates their walker or uses a flashy colored cane! Or I may be crabby and smack shins with the neon colored one.

I'm an only child, but had parents from large families—many relatives. Most of the family is gone now. The few remaining cousins either live far away or can't stand each other. I've remained neutral in this and have contact with two cousins on each side of the family. I have one son and I love him dearly. We get along well, have the same sense of humor and laugh a lot. He and his lovely wife live in another state although we see each other as often as we can. Their lives are busy and I don't see grandchildren in my future. One never knows so I suppose it could happen!

I live with my husband of 53 years. We eloped as teens and they said it wouldn't last. Guess we showed them. I had the good fortune of marrying into a family with wonderful people, each unique and I love them all. We have a family text chain that keeps us all in contact with each other daily. I look forward to the messages and pictures sent to me from my three sisters-in-law and their four daughters. Pictures of people or the latest flower in their garden are all welcome. The oldest of the nieces has just become a grandmother, lots of new baby pictures. Two others have children graduating from high school and one from college. I can live vicariously through them!

My job history starts with the usual retail job (sales clerk) while in high school and progressed to the waitress job in college, because they'll work with your class hours. I then went to office temp jobs. I next worked for a trucking company for six years at various positions from receptionist to head keypunch operator. (Note: Truckers will let you cross the picket line when you're the one who enters the info for their paychecks.) The first of my long-term jobs, 15 years as a sales/customer service rep for an international company. And my final job, 11 years, with many titles, including "Company Mom." All of these jobs had their merit, I made some friends along the way and I learned from each one. I think every kid should work in retail and one restaurant job if only to learn how to treat people and to see how these workers are treated too. I think I was the best at my last job because I felt appreciated, truly liked by my co-workers, and the pay was good. I sometimes miss my job, but I miss the people more.

Most of my early jobs did not pay well but I usually managed to save something even if it was only $5.00 to $10.00 a pay period. That doesn't sound like much now, but it adds up over time. I was raised with "If you can't pay cash for it, you don't need it." This wouldn't go over big now, but it made me very conscious of where my money was going. We haven't led an extravagant life or spent money we didn't have and it's paid off in the long run. Slow and steady wins the race and although we can't go crazy with spending, we're comfortable and that's all anyone really needs. I still buy the occasional lottery ticket though!

I would say I'm more spiritual than religious. Most organized religions are more of a business that acts in its own best interest than a group that's actually concerned with your soul. Religion, or man's interpretation of it, has done much harm over the centuries and the fact that we don't seem to be able to learn from that is worrisome.

I would like to think that something/someone, who is much smarter than man, is in control and eventually this world will get back on track. Although history does seem to keep repeating so I may be kidding myself. I HAVE lived long enough to have experienced some strange things that make me wonder if we aren't all connected in some way. There are definitely unexplainable occurrences from events in my life and the lives of others I know.

I would like to think there is some type of afterlife. I would also like to think there's such a thing as karma and that she pays special attention to politicians.

Random things I have learned along the way to becoming older:

Don't expect much and you will rarely be disappointed.

If you live long enough things just start growing on you. Sometimes overnight. Sometimes they disappear overnight. Magic?

Jim Morrison was right. People are *strange*.

The book was better.

Finally, my philosophy of life: I found this on the tag of a teabag from my hippie days in the 70's and it still applies: "*Things turn out best for those who make the best of the way things turn out.*"

2

7-11-46

Hi, here's a few lines for you, probably way too many lines. It's maybe a bit too personal, maybe much too long, but I hope it helps. I don't mean to be revealing too much, or boring you. It's just a can of worms subject, and I opened the can and this came out.

Like they say, this aging thing ain't for the faint of heart. At least that's what I think they said. My memory's seen better days. But it ain't that bad.

Emotionally, I'm a bit of a wreck. I tear up a lot and cry about stuff in these older years. Old times, phone calls from my granddaughter, a song I made up that resonates with me. Those kinds of things get me more than ever, and then the emotions flow. When a close friend dies, I hit the wall a bit. Start feeling an extra pain or two kicking in my side like a mule. I get emotional when I talk to my friend's wife, and am crying before even she is. I write something and I get emotional. My team wins the championship and I'm crying. Seems like my emotions are stronger than ever.

I like playing music and singing for kicks, but I take it seriously, really. Songs make me cry. The old gospel and blues stuff that hits deep does that to me. It has come more with age though it was here before. And I got plenty of that age thing. Emotions…always bubbling over for me.

A phone call from my grandson will do it, too. Of course, I think my grandkids should be phoning me more, and asking about my life, and treating me like their hero, the great wise man, but they aren't. They're too busy with their hand-held gadgets. So just hearing their voice puts me over. That's emotions for you.

Physically, I got a lot of pains here and there. Some bother me, and I wonder. Oh, No! Is it? Is it? THE BIG C? Am I having a heart attack? I got a couple of chest pains that are puzzling. Some of the pains shift from side to side. Makes me a little confused. I don't know what's ailing me. Kick in with Covid and I'm afraid to go to the doctor and find out. I think Covid kept me out of seeing my doctor, when I should have been.

I get afraid physically. Afraid to find out what those pains really are. But I walk most every day, and do stretches and some yoga in the morning and I feel good. Like I could live a long time. Hope I do. It's just the early morning monkey mind thing that drags me down. You shoulda' done this, or that, or shouldn't have said that to that guy 15 years ago, or last night. I know he's thinking about it. The monkeys keep getting bigger with age. I try to meditate, and I think it's working and then I'm climbing out of a rabbit hole again.

Yeah, Covid set me back. I think one of the biggest problems now for oldsters like me is dealing—and I mean all day long—with this crappy world run by technology. Don't call your doc, email her. Then she emails back. But with no details of the depth you inquired about. Take out some food? Sorry, we don't answer the phone. Try our app. Take a class in school. Got a tech application for you to fill out, and lots of security questions.

It's gotten too crazy. Tech has taken over, and that's not a strength of mine. I entered a Masters' program at state college, and every assignment is coupled with some kind of tech solution to turning in assignments. I write on paper, with a pen. Drives me nuts. There's a drop off in people my age going to my college. They're sick of all the tech, I'm told by someone who knows.

Then there's the lack of contact with old friends. Some die. Some get a little crazy, and aren't the same people. Fewer dear friends does not make this 70-something happy.

Covid did do something good for me. I have more time to write, and I'm writing the stories of my life and loving it even if it is hard as hell and I can't write that well. Taking college courses at 76 is interesting. The young kids and middle agers are cool to be around and they like having me in the class.

I spent many years as a newspaper man, and loved writing stories. So, I feel pretty good about myself. I can still write stories. Thanks to journalism for teaching me that. I'm glad I went into this field. It's got a lot of soul. Watch the noir movies about it. But the pay kind of sucked, so I still feel that.

Unfortunately, I had to leave my beloved San Francisco. Rents soared and I had to leave. I moved way down to a dusty Central Valley town. Big change. Big culture shift. Trying to adapt. Hotter than Hades. Not easy. But I'm making ends meet, just not sure which ends are meeting.

I feel pretty strong, really, despite aging, and Covid and the madness that consumed this country. I garden a lot, and spent a month or six weeks this summer picking figs, climbing up ladders. I have two fig trees, and I pick them for my friends. It makes me happy to give the figs to my fig-loving friends. One tree is as big as my garage, and I got hundreds and hundreds of figs from it.

As for my sex life, I still have one. A little more than occasionally it happens. And it feels great on a good night. My wife may not be as excited about it as I am, but she's up for it, and we have a good time. (Heading into the TMI zone.)

Swimming is my best exercise. I wish I had a pool. I would if I had made bigger bucks. It's hot out here where I had to move to make things more affordable.

But the job I had for years, a newspaper writer, was great. The money wasn't, so I rented a lot, and that became impossible. I did make enough to buy a house in the boondocks three years ago and I'm happy with the new pad.

I've got a family, with a brother and sister, a son, two grandchildren, a daughter-in-law, and I live with my lovely wife of more than 30 years and love her. She's the most important thing I have going. She's helping me live in these crazy times.

I never thought my country would go so far off the rails as to have nearly half the people supporting autocracy in the form of a criminal and insane person. He doesn't even believe in Democracy. This, for someone who is crashing deep into his '70s, is a nightmare of traumatic proportions. I hope I can survive this crazy state of affairs without slipping into insanity. Hope I'm not getting too dark. Obviously, these are times where truths like this are not often spoken freely and aloud.

Back on my job. I have loved being a journalist and I still do when I do it, but my life now is about taking this writing thing to another level, and that inspires me, despite my aches and pains and depression from aging and the state of the union. Things are very stressful now. With the emergence of people who dismiss the truth, or even can't accept that their candidate actually lost the election. This has become almost like the new dark ages. Very difficult on aging people who are dealing with their own physical health, mental health, etc.

Journalism? A resounding yes for me. To write a story and come in and see it in the paper the next day was a pure joy, and helped boost my self-esteem. I still love to write, and won't quit even if I don't finish my book of short stories. My wife and grandchildren want to read my next story on hopping freight trains from California to New Orleans, and that's inspiration enough to keep writing that story. Excuse the braggadociousness (is that a fucking word? It shouldn't be, and is misspelled if it is).

Newspapers did not put me in a "sittin' pretty" situation, and se la vi on that one. Journalism was worth it though, and gave me something I can take into this scary place of getting older. I may write about this aging disease when I finish the adventure stories.

Spiritually, I always liked the American Indians. They loved nature, the tribe, mother earth, the sun, the rivers, their water, the buffalo, wisdom, the land. I believe in all that stuff. Throw in some pop Buddhism and I feel the spirit. I'm still depressed. Tough to shake it in the current scene. But I continue reaching for the spirit. I don't need traditional religion. Seems like it's already wrecking the world we live in.

3

7-13-39

Lately, this past year, my feelings have been up and down because my husband's memory is declining and he's having some recurring medical problems. It's very hard to watch his frustration plus having to take on extra responsibilities that were his. Things like the finances, bill paying, etc. and securing workmen for home projects, etc.

My physical condition is good most of the time. I am fortunate to be my age and still be able to do the things I can. I take a couple of prescription meds but still do my housework, that is, cleaning, laundry, cooking (although I do find I don't enjoy planning and cooking meals as I once did). I still drive, thankful that I just renewed my driver's license. Yay! And I do not use a cane nor a walker.

We still occasionally have sex. (No further comment.)

We have three sons and two grandchildren. I live with my husband in our home that we purchased in 1973.

Before I was an Older, I worked as a "general" secretary for insurance adjusters. I enjoyed the people and the management who I worked with. I hope I was good at the job; I gave it my best. I do not miss working. I retired when the company left the area and my husband was also retiring. Do we ever make enough money?

Secure financially for now, thanks to a trusted broker. No mortgage.

I did not feel old until in my late 70s. Then I started to feel more slow in accomplishing tasks, etc. Also had more aches and pains and slower getting out of bed in the morning.

I am an only child and a native Texan. I am a Christian, am affiliated with a church and do believe in an afterlife.

What I'm finding is that everything is different now. Things fall apart one by one. Off to the doctor again and I'm not happy with that. But we're all going through it so I'm not alone.

4

12-9-36

How do I feel? It is difficult to describe. A little off in the head. A little forgetful, I lost nouns some time ago, light headed with loss of balance, generally okay. My doctors tell me I am unusually fit for a woman of my age. I believe that is in part because I was always physically active and played tennis into my 70s. I often feel bored, like there's not enough to keep me occupied. And I also feel a bit helpless.

I think this is one of the worst times of my life…not my life but the world's life. Ukraine's people being cruelly slaughtered. The climate crisis being all but ignored so the fossil fuel industry can keep making gazillions of bucks, and the pandemic that took about two years out of our lives and the complete lives lost for millions of people worldwide. And now our SCOTUS has abandoned Roe v. Wade, the proscription for safe medical care for any of the desperate women who need it. All the women my age will remember the dangerous ways women sought to end their pregnancies before R v. W. Women were dying and will die again now that this actually happened.

No one likes abortion. Some pregnancies come from horrible circumstance or at a time in a woman's life when she cannot abide trying to care for and pay for a child. I got pregnant the first time I was intimate with a young man, at age 18. My elder sister explained how we could arrange an abortion… but that was not for me. So having a child changed the direction of my life especially compared to other women my age. I went to 6 different undergraduate schools before I got my B.A. at age 34. And at age 44 I received my Ph.D. All this during two husbands and three children. The children being the way most important thing I did in my whole life.

I have never experienced any time that had all terrible things going on at once. Again, I feel a bit helpless.

A couple weeks ago we had some Older friends in for lunch. We talked about ain't it awful and wished we could do something about it. I suggested we, the four of us, march to Washington. It was good for a laugh. No one really thought it was a good idea. In the past I have seen news stories about Older people, women mostly, hiking along the highway to faraway places to make a statement about the Vietnam War or some other terrible thing that was going on.

My physical condition as I said, is probably pretty good, yet…I went for a routine dental appointment, teeth cleaning…oops, I had to go to the oral surgeon to have one of my teeth extracted from which a filling had departed. Then I went to get new glasses, which I hadn't done for several years partly because of the pandemic…oh, no glasses for you. You have to go for cataract surgery (this surgery was a few weeks ago and it was no easy feat, though everyone told me it would be). I go for a routine bone density test, yep, I have osteoporosis. The doctor suggested I not fall down…duh! March 2022 marked the five years that had passed since my breast cancer. So, one by one, little parts of our bodies deteriorate and become useless. And the little pain here and the big pain there become more frequent. And probably like many old women, in the night, I sometimes don't make it to the bathroom fast enough as the pee trickles down my leg.

Back to the cataract surgery. I see things that I never saw, one being the abundance of lines and sags in my face. I look many years older than I thought I did and my lifelong vanity took a twang. Things are a different color. Everything is bathed in a white sort of light. Before, the cataracts were kind of like always wearing unprescribed sun glasses.

All that said, I do not use a cane nor a walker and I take one regular medicine for heart arrhythmia that I have had all my life. I am told that Olders usually have an extensive list of medicines for this, that, and the other thing. I take many vitamins and supplements. I ride the stationary bike 30 minutes each day at the lowest, easiest rate. So generally, I am okay.

No sex for many years. Husband's earlier prostate cancer one of the main reasons.

I have two grown children who themselves each have two nearly grown children. I am proud of all of them. They are smart, industrious, accomplished, and wonderful. No great-grandchildren. My children are from very solicitous and concerned to "I really don't care what's happening in your life." When Ellie was here, I never thought our children paid enough attention to her. Her husband, whom she didn't like very much anyway, had passed away some years ago. So, she, unlike me, was very alone.

I know, our children have their own lives to attend to. But I'm thinking the Asians and others have it right that the family stays together into old age. The Olders there are constantly surrounded with family so don't experience the isolation as much as it is felt by Olders in this country. It is a huge treat to have a phone call or a drop by from one of my children or grandchildren.

I have a small olive oil business. For several years we owned the orchard which was seven hours away by car. We sold oil at ten local farmers' markets. After we got too tired and old for that, we sold the orchard and sell now primarily to people who know us from farmers markets and from the cart on our website. It is an excellent product and we're proud of it.

Prior to that I spent years working in non-profits and state-run health organizations. In the seventies my then husband and I founded and operated a non-profit, live-in treatment program for young addicts, runaways, and dropouts. I did this for about 10 years. Very gratifying, fun and interesting. I worked as Exec Director for a battered women's shelter, then for many years helped people quit smoking working for the public health department. I wrote a book about quitting.

And I wrote other books. One of my husbands was a football coach. I would sit in the stands with the other gals who had no idea what was going on. So, of course, I wrote the book to help women understand and enjoy the game of football. From my experience at the live-in treatment center, I also wrote a book about parenting. I wrote one movie script based on the memoires of a fisher lady. And here I am now, writing this.

Do I feel how I spent my productive years was important? I do. I must have helped hundreds of people quit smoking which is life-saving. I was also interested in the political goings on and when I could I participated in local politics. I think one of my biggest regrets is that I never actually ran for political office. Before there were any female county Board of Supervisors members, I seriously considered running for that office…but never did. It seemed to me that politicians spent much of their time in meetings, which is how I spent much time working for public health and it got tiresome. That said, the work I did with people was in some cases lifesaving so that was good.

The money I made was of little consequence. If I really needed something my parents were always willing to share even though my father, a civil servant, was not a wealthy man. I have never felt poor or in need.

One of the happiest times of my life was when I was on a spiritual path. My grown son, who was ill with AIDS, directed me to that place. He was into crystals which for some spiritualists carry different energies. One day after he passed I found a pink crystal lying in the yard. No explanation as to where it might have come from. Pink crystals are associated with love. Of course, I believed it was somehow from him.

I went to lectures about and read and practiced issues in "A Course In Miracles." I recommend it. As time went on, I went away from it to other things. Spirituality needs to be nurtured and practiced to maintain. I do love music of all sorts, learned piano from my gramma at age five and sang in the Sunday School choir. I believe music to be the highest form of human endeavor…by highest I mean spiritually.

And one of the most delightful things in my life is the internet. I was in my 40s when I was researching to write my doctorate. I went to the university library and poured through all those little recipe cards finding what I needed to read. Now one goes to the internet with any question and an answer will be forthcoming. I love, love, love it. There is nothing I can't learn about. If I were to advise Olders about how to make life a bit more tolerable I would say, get a tablet, get Google and go for information acquiring or play solitaire or write a book. If you can't do it by yourself, get someone to help you.

And I watch sports. I'm a big Angels fan. I quit the Dodgers because I couldn't get them on TV where we live. I like the Clippers and the Rams. My husband and I have a role reversal. He's in the living room watching movies and I'm in the bedroom watching whatever sports team is currently playing.

And I would not be being honest if I did not mention that not infrequently, the question comes to mind, how much longer do I have? Inside I feel much younger than I am but will I be gone tomorrow or next year or what? One of the things that keeps bringing that up is this Health Care Directive that we're all supposed to do. Part of it is what do you want when you die. I said to my children they could decide. Whatever was easiest for them. But no, they insist I decide what I want to happen to my leftovers when I leave. So, what do I want? Who knows?

5

3-27-47

How do I feel emotionally? It varies day to day. Some days are good, but others are rough. I had to retire 3 years ago from a job that I loved. My health declined to a point where I could no longer perform my duties to an acceptable level. I was in my job for over 17 years. For 16 out of 17 years my yearly performance evaluations were "Exceptional." But my 17th year proved to be a disaster. Emotional problems in my family, along with a significant decline in my health caused me to voluntarily retire. This was very hard for me. People at the job would always ask me "When are you going to retire?" My answer was—"When they carry me out of here." They didn't have to carry me out. In concert with my lovely and wise wife, I cleaned out my office and slowly and humbly walked out. It was over.

I almost immediately slipped into depression. It became very difficult to get out of bed. I no longer had a purpose. I realized that like many men I counted on my job for my purpose, my identity, and self-esteem. Without my job I found myself quickly slipping into the void.

Also, I had been the bread winner in my family for over 30 years. In a flash I went from a very respectable income to Social Security and a couple of meager pensions. I was far from destitute, but I could no longer buy or do what I wanted when I wanted. As my daughter would say, "This is a 1st world problem." As one of my friends would say, "Be grateful for what you have." Excellent advice.

Roles in my family changed in a heartbeat. My wife suddenly became the breadwinner. That was hard for me, and my wife. She had to shoulder the major responsibility for paying the mortgage and keeping us in our home. She never complains. She works very hard at a difficult job. The saving grace is that she loves her job. I love her to the moon and back.

My physical condition? I have struggled through several health challenges. In 2015 I suffered a stroke.

I owe my life to our cat. She wakes us up at 5AM each day for us to feed her. She jumps up on the bed and hits me in the head with her paw to wake me up…true. On that fateful morning I got out of bed with a terrible headache and vertigo. I tried to pull myself together and went downstairs to feed her. I felt something was wrong when I found myself spilling cat food all over the kitchen floor. Next, I tried tying my shoe. I couldn't do it. It was then that I realized that this was more than a bad headache. It was one of those moments when you say to yourself, "I can't screw around. I've got to get to the hospital. I'm having a stroke."

I didn't want to freak out my wife who at times is very excitable. I tried to stay calm cause I needed her to drive me to the ED. I went back upstairs. I said to her, "This vertigo is horrible. I think you need to take me to Cedars ED."

Along with the wake-up kitty, we had a dog who now needed to go out. My wife said, "Ok but I'm not taking that damn dog out." I went back downstairs and got the leash. As I was fastening it to the dog's harness, he looked at me with a puzzled expression that said, "What is wrong with you?" All my life I believed that critters are very sensitive. He knew what was going on. I took him out. He did his business then wife and I got in the car and were off.

She drove me to the hospital. When we got there, I calmly said to the admitting doctor, "I believe I am having a stroke." At that point my wife almost fainted.

"Why didn't you tell me?"

I responded, "I didn't want to worry you."

I was very lucky. There was a neurologist in the ED. She told us that she was conducting a study on a drug called a clot buster. I said, "Give it to me!"

She responded, "I must tell you that it could cause an internal bleed in your head. That is the downside." I asked her what she would do if I refused the drug. She said, "We would give you an aspirin and put you on the ward."

And I immediately replied…"Give me that drug." It turned out to be wonderful. It stopped the stroke in its tracks. But I do have some residual problems. The clot was on the left side of my brain, so it affected my right side. I used to pride myself on my handsome handwriting. After the stroke my writing was more like chicken scratches. I also have slight limp on my right side and my balance is horrible. No more motorcycles for me, one of my great loves.

Then after that I had bilateral hip replacement. Then major surgery on my lower back which entailed putting a metal bracket to separate discs. My surgeon described what he was doing as no problem. That made me laugh. I said I'm becoming more and more bionic by the day. In 2021 I had 3 stents placed in my heart. There were several more minor events to add to these major ones.

After the back surgery I had to add a cane to my daily life. This was another challenge that I had to get used to. I flinched when my doctor suggested a cane to help me with balance issues. "I'm a man, God damnit, I am very adept at navigating on my own." Nonetheless, after falling down a few times it was either purchase a helmet or use the cane. I found the cane very helpful.

And who was I in my younger years? An actor.

I do miss it on occasion. I really loved it. I had a great time. I always looked forward to going to work each day. I must correct that statement. I never considered acting as work even though the physical and emotional demands were difficult at times. Also, the uncertainty of down time between employment was always worrying. There was always the nagging fear—"Will I ever work again?" and it was a slim existence financially.

However, I am proud to say that for years I was part of a small group of actors (10% of my Union—Actors Equity Association) that could boast they made a living solely as an Actor. I was so fortunate to perform most all the time. I am very proud of what I was able to achieve. Shakespeare wrote 34 plays and I performed in 28 of 34. In a single 4-year period I performed in 24 plays. That's 6 plays a year (4 plays in Cleveland, and 2 in San Diego). I commuted between Cleveland and San Diego twice a year on my motorcycle. It was a wonderful time!

I loved my trips between San Diego and Cleveland, and back again. I love the open road, and I loved crossing the country on my motorcycle. It's a whole different experience than being in a car. A car is nice, but your view of the country is framed by the windshield. It's like watching the country go by on TV. On a bike the experience is 360 degrees. You are experiencing the country full on. Whatever the weather, wind, rain, sleet, snow, hot, cold, you are in the middle of what is happening, and to me that was exhilarating! I should also mention that I believe the reason people love motorcycles is in the "way it moves you." After hours on the road, the bike becomes an extension of your body; enough so that at times, you are so connected you feel yourself moving through space detached from all restrictions of space and time. Fantastic!

I never pursued acting expecting to be a Star. My goal from the beginning was to be a "working" actor playing the Classics. I loved Shakespeare in particular. I was happy working in Regional Theatre. I graduated from theatre school at a time when there was a blossoming of Regional Theatres across the country. The hope and promise were that there would be a Professional Company in every major city. An actor could go from town to town practicing his craft playing the Classics. That sounded like heaven to me.

For years I was able to make my dream a reality. I worked and played leading roles with major Theatre Companies across the Country. I acted multiple seasons with the Oregon Shakespeare Festival, The Old Globe Theatre in San Diego, The San Diego Rep, The Denver Center Theatre Company, The Alaska Rep in Anchorage Alaska, and for years I was a member of the Resident Acting Company at the Cleveland Play House.

Working at the Play House was an honor as it was the first permanent Professional Theatre Company in the United States. It was founded in 1916. It was at the Play House that I had the opportunity to work with playwright, Arthur Miller on a new play of his titled THE ARCHBISHOP'S CEILING. My last show at the Play House was a play titled BILLY BISHOP GOES TO WAR. It was a two actor play about the most decorated Canadian Aviator in WWI. That show was the most challenging part in my career. I worked with a piano player and played 19 characters and had to sing and dance.

I met my wife onstage. We were playing opposite each other in a production of LOVES LABORS LOST at the Old Globe Theatre in San Diego. I played the clown, Costard, and she played the country girl love interest. I should also mention that we got married on Christmas Eve morning in 1988. We were married at 9 am at her sister's house in San Juan Capistrano. By noon we had to hurry back to San Diego because I was playing Scrooge in CHRISTMAS CAROL at the San Diego Rep and had two shows that day.

After marrying we moved to LA. We were living with my mother-in-law. My wife did very well with TV and Commercials. I was a lost soul, a fish out of water. I could not connect/relate to the LA scene. I was used to working all the time. In LA actors do a spot on TV or film. Then it seemed to me that they go to lunch until the next job comes along. I got a lot of auditions when I first got here but ended up blowing all of them. I was not used to auditioning (terrible nerves) and my acting style was too big. I could not adjust to playing to the camera.

Prior to coming to LA, I never had to audition. I knew a lot of people and had a great reputation. I would get phone calls offering me work, and I would either take the job or not. The final straw came after meeting with an agent. She asked me, "What do you do?"

I responded in all humility saying, "What do you need?" (Remember, prior to coming to LA I did BILLY BISHOP playing 19 roles.) Well, she got very angry, and ended the interview.

I was really depressed after that incident. Then I get a phone call from The Alabama Shakespeare Festival offering me a Season playing great roles and offering me good money. I was excited. I immediately told my wife. She was not impressed.

She said, "Great. That means that you are going back on the road. I thought you wanted to settle down and raise a family? How are we going to maintain a relationship with you on the road?"

I agreed. I called the Artistic Director and said, "Thank you for thinking of me, but I just got married, and need to stay in LA."

She was right. I told her I thought it would be best if I got a job and she agreed. That led me to getting a job at Samuel French, the oldest playwright representative Agent in the country. They hired me to work in the Accounting Department doing Accounts Receivable. When I started, they asked me if I knew anything about computers? I had just completed a beginning class on IBM Computers, so I told them "Oh yeah."

"Are you familiar with Apple Computers?"

I told them, "No, but I am certain I can learn quickly."

They said, "OK." That was the beginning of a new adventure.

And now, you see, in my head I'm 25 years old. In reality I am 75. I decided that if I am going to continue with this journey I had to adjust. I made the adjustment, and I'm happy to report that I am doing just fine even without motorcycles or acting.

And now to Spirituality.

This is a complex topic for me. I hope I can make some sense out of it. Here goes. At 75 looking back over the years I find myself spending more and more time focused on Spirituality. Maybe it's because I have arrived at the last quarter of my life. Who knows. I'm just now beginning to realize my

Spirituality has been built upon an eclectic number of random "peak" experiences/blessings which re-enforce my belief in a higher power. My life has been and continues to be a game of "Lost and Found."

My hero, Zen Philosopher, Alan Watts states that the first game a baby learns is lost & found. For example—As a baby lying in a cradle or crib you find yourself looking at your mother. She is looking back at you in a loving manner. You are peaceful, content. All is right with the world. Then suddenly, she places her hands in front of her face. To you she appears to have disappeared. She is gone. You feel lost. You cry out. Then suddenly she takes her hands away—Peekaboo! Once lost, now found. My life, as most others, has taken a lot of twists and turns, and lost and found experiences, which are now finally beginning to make sense to me.

I was raised Catholic, but over the years I have come to relate more with the principles of Zen Buddhism. Some people refer to a person who maintains this philosophy as a "Cabu," a Catholic Buddhist. My parents were devout Catholics. They instilled in me a strong belief and importance of a Spiritual life. They never missed Mass on Sunday. I was an Altar Boy from age 8 to age 13.

I served 6 o'clock Mass in the morning for an old Polish Priest. His name was Father Jarosz. He was a good man. He was gassed in WWI which severely damaged his lungs. He would often experience some outrageous coughing fits during Mass. This did not scare me. My heart always went out to him. I would remain quiet and motionless until he could regain his composure. When he was able, we picked up where we left off. I served Mass for him for years. I never missed. He was a special man. He didn't talk much, and he never expressed any outward emotions, but I knew instinctively that he was a significant individual and that he liked me.

I loved the peace and quiet of the church at that time of the morning. It was empty except for a few old ladies and the Nuns from the school. It was a very special space and time: Holy Grounds. Quiet. Quiet. When I look back on it, I realize I was caught up deeply with the theatricality and ritual of the service. It was my introduction to meditation.

However, by the age of 18 I began to have serious doubts. My faith began to waver as I experienced more and more incongruities in the church. For example, when I was 18, I volunteered as a Lecture (a person who leads prayers during the Mass). I remember being in the Sacristy (the room behind the altar where the priest prepares for Mass). One day while waiting for the Mass to begin I overheard a conversation between the Pastor of the church (a very bigoted man) and one of the Parishioners who sold Real Estate. It was a very heated discussion during which I heard the Pastor say—"I don't want you selling any more homes to Mexicans."

The church was located in a heavily Spanish speaking community. I couldn't believe my ears. Yet, it made perfect sense to me. It confirmed in my mind that there was a definite difference between the religion and the people representing the religion. Shortly after that encounter and others too numerous to mention, I stopped going to church. I couldn't cope with the hypocrisy.

It was that incident and more like it (the constant plea for more and more money, etc.). Now this didn't mean that I stopped believing in God, or a higher power, no not at all. For me, the people representing the religion often got in the way and gave the religion a bad name.

My quitting didn't go over well with my parents. They were furious when I refused to go to church. They couldn't drive, so were dependent on me to take them. I was happy to drive them there, drop them off, and pick them up after the service. It was an uneasy compromise.

The most important Holiday in Catholicism is Easter. No matter what, every Catholic is bound to go to Communion on Easter and renew their vows to God and the church. Well, one day right before Easter I was at home when everyone else in the house was gone. My mother needed to go to Confession before Easter. She asked me to take her.

I drove her to the church and told her that I would pick her up later. She was adamant—"You are going to Confession!" I loved my mother dearly and couldn't refuse her. At the same time, I was angry. I didn't believe in Confession, but at the same time did not want to just go through the motions and disrespect the priest. It was a dilemma.

I found myself in line at the Confessional. When it was my time I entered the Confessional, but I was not going to go against my beliefs. Instead of kneeling down, I sat down on the Kneeler. What was I going to do? When the priest slid the window open to indicate he was ready to hear my confession. Instead of saying the usual "Bless me father for my sins, my last confession was…" There was a long pause. I finally said, "Hi." The priest was taken aback, but to my surprise he was very understanding. I explained the situation with my mother and didn't want to offend her. At the same time, I didn't want to disrespect him. I explained that along the way I had behaved in a manner that would easily qualify as sins. However, I believed that I had learned a great deal about myself.

We talked and talked, and finally I said, "Father, I've been here quite a while. I should go. There are other people waiting to see you." Matter of fact there was an old gentleman that twice opened the door and closed it quickly seeing me sitting on the kneeler. He was shocked. I could see it in his face.

The priest said, "Let me give you a blessing before you go."

I said, "Great."

Also, he said, "Why don't you stop by the rectory some time. I enjoyed our talk and would like to continue our conversation."

I said "OK." When I finally walked out of the confessional all the people in line looked at me as though I was the biggest sinner of all time. My mom just smiled.

As I mentioned earlier, I consider myself to be spiritual. Spirituality holds an important place in my life. It always has, though I am not connected with any formal religion. My faith is grounded in

Nature, and all God's creatures. When I am at the beach or in the mountains, or even in my backyard feeding the birds or squirrels I am in church. I'm meditating. I must admit the older I get the more of a sucker I am for all of God's creatures.

I believe in an afterlife. I don't know exactly what it is. However, I'm pretty sure it is not what most people call "Heaven." I get the sense that many people feel that once in Heaven, all their suffering is ended, and they are forever happy. How boring is that! Nor, do I believe there is a Hell. I believe Hell is here on earth. Everyone experiences Hell many times throughout their life. I believe Evil is a reality. It comes in many forms. It is a sickness. There are evil people. They are not devils, but I believe their evil behavior is a sickness: a mental illness.

There are some people I call "Psychic Vampires." They present themselves as nice, ordinary people. They are attracted to kind, sensitive people. However, after spending time with them, suddenly, they attach themselves to you and suck the life out of you. They take advantage of you, exhaust you, and leave you very unhappy. It takes a while to recognize these people, but once you do, you clear out fast.

My personal philosophy had been heavily influenced by the teachings of the Zen Philosopher Alan Watts. At one time he was an Episcopal Bishop. I don't have this phrase totally correct; however, I believe he said something like, "It is said that Religion is a boat to carry us across the river to the ultimate reality/Spirituality." Once you arrive there, there is no need to go back. You got it. Alan states that people spend much of their lives going back and forth across the river from Religion to Spirituality and back again.

Spirituality is a state of mind. Please understand I hope I don't sound like I'm boasting that I am something "special" in my awareness. I am just "regular" like everyone else. I have so many lessons yet to learn. When people ask me about my Spirituality, I simply say—"I'm just a pilgrim on the road."

I am not afraid of dying. I have been close to death many times on my motorcycle, so it is not strange or scary to me. In my last job as a Palliative Care Social Worker, I have been blessed to be present at many deaths. I view dying as a uniquely sacred process specific to everyone.

A caution to the reader, please understand the description that follows is not Scientific. It is my own understanding and knowledge of the Dying

Process. To me it mirrors the birthing process, although in reverse. (Also, it precludes sudden death, which in and of itself is a particular situation.) The final phase for many individuals begins when the person is near death and appears to go in and out of consciousness. They enter a sort of "no man's land." They are not in this world, and not yet in the other.

A certain definite circular rhythm begins. At one point the person appears to be passing, then just before it looks as though the person is dead, then the process stops and reverses itself. They return to a somewhat normal rhythm. My own name for this process is "hooking up." There is no specific time limit to this process. It can occur over a period of minutes or stretch to weeks. I believe it is when all the roadblocks or personal issues that are holding them back/keeping them in this world are resolved. When that happens, the person lets go and dies.

After the passing all that remains is an empty shell. Looking at the body there is no question that the person is no longer there. The spirit has moved on. To where… Who knows. In my mind they are beginning a new adventure. They are free. As Shakespeare would say, "they are free of this mortal coil."

Sometimes prior to passing on, the patient will wait until a loved one keeping vigil will leave the room. This often causes despair to the person keeping vigil. They mistakenly blame themselves for leaving the room, when that is just what the patient was waiting for. Their wish was to die alone.

I believe in Guardian Angels. Once again, please know that I do not consider myself special. We all have them. Mine have been with me all my life. They have protected me many times during my crazy life. For example, one time occurred in 1972 while I was hitchhiking from Detroit to San Jose. One blazing morning in June, I found myself standing on an onramp, next to a lamp post on I-80. I was headed West. The signpost on the freeway read Little America, Wyoming. In my head I thought, where the hell is that? I was exhausted, and in the middle of nowhere. I hadn't slept in two days. I just got off a Semi I had been riding on through the night. I had no idea where I was in the country. All I had was $30 dollars in my pocket and warm water in my canteen. I was fleeing a broken marriage, and I was "shit out of luck." You could say—I was way out on the edge.

To complicate matters further I was wearing Electric Green Pants. My life was Surreal at the time, and every person or situation I encountered was another scene. To top it off I was holding a cardboard sign indicating that I was headed to the NORTH POLE. How ridiculous. Who is going to pick this clown up?

I knew that I needed to get a ride, pronto. I couldn't wait around. I was in the desert, and it was going to get unbearably hot in a few hours. I had a lot of experience hitch-hiking. I learned that the key to getting a ride was to quickly establish a connection with the oncoming car. As soon as they came into sight I would focus on the driver's eyes, sending the psychic message, "Please pick me up. I'm OK. Friendly/harmless and I desperately need a ride." It worked. After about a half hour, a car pulled over. I quickly approached the passenger window. To my shock and pleasant surprise, the driver turned out to be my friend, David. I knew him from Detroit. We were students the previous year in the Graduate Theatre Program at Wayne State University.

How did this happen? I believe my Guardian Angel must have been working overtime. You see, when the Semester ended, David was going to an Acting Job in Florida. While there he got very sick. David's home was in Reno. His father drove to Florida to bring David home. David told me that

20 minutes before seeing me he had been asleep in the back seat of the car. When he saw me, he told his dad to pull over. Lucky me. David said, smilingly, "There is only one person in the world I knew that would be hitch-hiking in those pants."

Another time on one of my cross-country motorcycle adventures my Guardian Angel saved me from going down at high speed in the rain. I was headed East to Cleveland on I-70 in Kansas. The weather was horrible. I had been riding in the rain for three days. Miserable. It was about 11 am just about 50 miles West of Kansas City.

Kansas is generally flat. Flat. Flat. However, this part of the state is rolling hills. I hadn't been on the road very long when I crested a hill and was on my way down the other side. When I got to the bottom of the hill the road was flooded and my bike began to hydroplane.

I was losing control of the bike and could feel it listing to the left on the way over. At that crucial moment I screamed, "No. Son of a bitch!" And pulled the bike back and regained control. I was so scared I nearly messed my pants. I was breathing heavily.

Once I caught my breath, I decided that this was an Omen—You are not supposed to be on the road today. I pulled off at the next exit and got a motel room. Enough. I rode nothing but a motorcycle for 13 years, and this was the first time in all those years I was close to crashing. "Thank you, Jesus, and my Guardian Angel."

6

12-29-36

How do I feel? At my age of 85 I feel fortunate to basically feel very good. Emotionally I am definitely happy, satisfied, inspired, and sensitive. Physically I feel good and healthy for the most part. How do I feel about myself? I would say I am happy, cheerful, compassionate, affectionate, and I have a love for God, family, and friends. Also, I have an extreme love for all animals and the beauty of nature.

My physical condition is reasonably good. I do have a few non-life-threatening conditions which I have to watch closely and make sure I take my medications, exercise, and see my doctors regularly. These conditions are: osteoarthritis, osteoporosis, high blood pressure, and my kidneys are beginning to show signs of decreased function. But my doctor says I am reasonably stable.

As far as sexual activity is concerned, I was still active up to and until my husband became ill and passed away at the age of 73 after 54 years of marriage. Since then, I no longer engage in sexual activity which I attribute to my personal and religious beliefs.

I do not use a cane, walker, or wheel chair yet. My balance is a little shaky since I broke my fibula. Consequently, I am very careful walking and going up and down stairs. Since I do have osteoporosis, I need to be extra careful.

I have lots of family. I have outlived all of my family who I grew up with. (My parents, my older brother, and all of my aunts and uncles.) I married young, at 18, my husband was 19. We had our first child almost four years later. We had a total of five children: four sons and one daughter. All five were born healthy. We were very fortunate. Family vacations was one of our greatest joys. We loved to travel.

All five of our children graduated from college. This was one of our dreams, since neither my husband nor I did. All five are married and still married to their original spouses. Therefore, we have been blessed with 18 grandchildren and so far, 13 great grandchildren.

I no longer live alone. After seven years of being alone after my husband's passing away, my daughter and her husband invited me to move in with them. They felt it would help me financially and they wouldn't have to keep checking in on me. After much consideration we all agreed it would be best. They have the room to give me my own bedroom and bathroom. It has worked out well. I am still able to help with cooking and housework. Also, I know I have help if or when I need it.

Before becoming an Older, I was busy being a wife, raising a family, was active in my church, and worked in banking. I only had one year of college and wasn't enjoying it, so the banking job was blessing and it turned out to be my occupation for years. Eventually we moved to another state to get away from the smog. At that point I was able to stay home to take care of my children. What a blessing that was for me and my family. When my youngest was old enough to attend school, I took a part-time job at the local bank. That eventually turned into a full-time job.

While the work was fulfilling, worthwhile, and definitely necessary I do not miss it. I worked 36 years and was still able to be at home when my family needed me. I finally retired at age 76.

I would say I was good at what I did. I wish I had realized earlier that accounting and computers were what I was good at, I may have finished college. But events in my life led me in this direction. It was a time when banks were converting from hand posting, etc., to computers, so it was a challenge, which I enjoyed very much. I was eventually promoted to head of the bookkeeping and tellers, and was promoted to be an officer in the bank.

I felt that I was well paid with my banking job. It included a very nice Christmas bonus. But today it wouldn't be enough. Also, I should include that the bank owners decided to sell to a larger bank which made us only a small branch. As a result, I was out of a job because of "downsizing." I was very upset as I had given them an excellent 20 years of my life. They let the higher paid employees go so they could hire younger ones for less money. That was difficult to accept but I held my head high. I was 62 so I took early retirement.

I stayed home for a few years looking for other work until a friend asked me to come work in their family-owned business. I became their receptionist and accountant. I managed the deposits, paid bills, and did the payroll. I worked another 10 years for them and it was very satisfying.

All in all, I feel I have had a fulfilling life, but 36 years of work outside the home was enough.

And now, financial considerations are an issue. My husband didn't have a nice retirement plan as he was a farmer for the majority of his life. But I had a food profit-sharing retirement from my last bank. I have planned well; I am totally debt free. I was able to save a good amount from the sale of my house. My final death expenses are taken care of so my children won't have to come up with that expense when I am gone. I pay my daughter an agreed amount of rent for taking care of me. Also, I am able to pay all the health insurances that I need. I do all of this out of my Social Security and some left over for other incidental expenses. And I have my savings for an emergency.

About my religion: yes, it is very important to me. I can't remember a time that my family didn't attend and participate in church regularly. I grew up in a Community Church. When I married, we continued as a couple but at his church for convenience. Religion has been a big part of my life. Especially while we were raising our family. It was important to give thanks before meals, to talk about what it means to love Christ. That comes from the home. As an Older I feel it's more important than ever.

I am concerned about what is happening to our churches today. So many are splitting because of liberal and conservative political differences. I am struggling a bit over all this. I want a church that preaches "The Truth" from the Bible. I have found one but I have to watch it on-line because it is too far away to attend. I supplement watching that with reading my Bible, doing devotions and praying daily, and listening to Christian music.

"I can do all things through Christ who strengthens me." Philippians 4:13.

7

2-28-39

How do I feel? Ok, but less than perfect. Growing old and living alone has its challenges. Emotionally, I would like to find someone to share my life with, but that's a challenge and I don't know how to solve that problem. How do I feel physically? I have several ailments, none immediately life threatening. I am able to walk and talk and even try Pickle Ball, carefully, but I can no longer pilot an aircraft. I'm OK, but I have moments when I miss my wife who died two years ago. One thing that I am proud of is that I cared for her at home until the end. That's what she wanted and I was able to do that. I actually miss being able to care for her.

Describing my physical condition is not so easy. Peripheral neuropathy, varicose veins, balance issues, slight tick in my heart, and short-term memory loss. But I am able to walk for maybe two miles and I try to play PB being careful not to fall. I have fallen a few times with bumps and bruises but no broken bones. I use no cane nor walker. (And about 2 months after I wrote this, I was in the hospital for bypass surgery following a mild heart attack.)

Sexually active? How about never. I attempted to have intercourse with my wife maybe six years ago but it was very painful for her so that stopped immediately. And none since. I doubt that I could get an erection at this point…but I'd like to try.

About family, yes, I have three children and four grandchildren. And I live alone. One of my thoughts and concerns is dying alone and not being discovered until the police arrive days later.

What did I do before becoming old and how do I feel about it now? I'm convinced now that I spent too many years in Graduate School hanging around academia. I must also add that during that time I got a Ph.D. and a Lifetime Post-Secondary Education Teaching Credential. When I finally quit doing that and took a full-time job it was with the Federal Government in Washington, D.C. with the FAA. I have been officially retired for 28 years. In retrospect it worked out okay but not at all what I imagined or was even capable of imagining. I think now that I made more than one career mistake.

That said, I worked in a large office but I really enjoyed field work. I think that I did a good job and that the work that we did was important. I don't miss working in D.C. Even though I live less than an hour away from my old office, I have visited the building that I worked in just twice since retirement 28 years ago.

I was good at what I did and worked my way up to regional branch manager covering a large piece of the country. Again, I certainly could have made better career choices. Money was never an issue for me and I made enough to live on and raise a family.

I owned and flew my own airplane and had Commercial Pilot and Flight Instructor ratings. Flying is nearly an existential experience; every takeoff absolutely demands a successful landing. No exceptions. To plan and execute a flight demands a high skill level and there is satisfaction in knowing that you have that skill…a dream of mankind for thousands of years. There is a great feeling of freedom as you rise above the ground and you see more and more of the world around you as it exists and you rise in the sky and finally see a horizon. That's very satisfying.

I enjoyed flying solo more than carrying passengers. Flight instruction was fun, students varied in learning ability and it was a challenge to prep and teach the next lesson. It required dedication to learn to fly, expensive in both cost and time, but the rewards were special. And yes, I miss it but have no regrets.

And now about finances, I live month to month but in retirement my income is greater than the US average for a family of four in California, greater than $60K. Really, I don't see how a family can live on that. I also have some savings and most importantly, great health insurance. I am a Disabled Veteran so that helps.

Do I have religion and an afterlife? No life after death as in there is no fountain of youth. We are all a piece and part of the galaxy called the Milky Way. I think that the idea of an afterlife has a stronger pull on us as we age…we are getting closer to the final exit and wouldn't it be nice if our loved ones were there to greet us. Nah, but that said, I have felt something like the presence a couple times from each of the wives I lost. Hmmm.

What else should our readers know about me? What I would like them to know that too, too often we take our spouses for granted. It is not intentional, it is just life, like the air we breathe, that he or she will always be there. That the meals will be prepared, the laundry done, the clothes deposited at the dry cleaners, the home neat, clean, and organized. We feel there will always be enough money and that life will be forever worry free. Then your spouse dies and the world changes. That has happened to me twice. Additionally, moving around the country, chasing the next promotion, leaving your home town has a cost. It is sometimes lonely in a foreign land.

8

4-9-46

How do I feel emotionally? Well, it depends on what day it is. Some days, things are going well, everything is falling into place, and I am at peace with the world. Other days, I deal with recalcitrant clients, my neighbors' dogs won't stop barking, and I have to figure out a way to explain to my wife that I have to travel to some faraway place that she does not want to a) go to, b) does not want me to go to, or c) decides that it is not a good place for anyone to go to.

I count myself fortunate to be working at a job that I love, doing work that I am really good at, and continuing to be productive at an age when most men are retired, lost in dementia, or gone. I know that there is a stigma attached to the "grind" of working until you drop, but that is my dream. I have no desire to be "retired" and simply do nothing, waiting to leave this mortal coil. I want to keep doing my work until I can't do it any longer.

My financial situation is stable, and I have enough money to live out my life. However, I did not really start thinking about an end game early on. My early days in the business of theatre and television were spent as an actor, singer, dancer, stage manager, freelance designer, and finally as a consultant, designing and engineering performance technical systems for Theatres, TV Studios, and Sound Stages.

I traveled a lot, lived simply with few possessions and had some of the best experiences of my life. I met some very creative and fun people to work with, experienced the excitement of being part of something much bigger than little ol' me, creating events that entertained, challenged, and maybe even got some people thinking about things. In my travels, I experienced the way many different people live their lives, in very different cultures, but I found that most people are the same: we all want to love and be loved, to contribute, to make a difference, and be allowed to live as we choose.

I am concerned that I may lose my brain functions and turn into a carrot. I can live with losing 10 seconds on the 40-yard dash, not being able to bench press my weight, or not being as sexy as my shirt, but if I cannot be sentient, put two and two together, do my work, well, that would be a major kick in the head. If and when that time comes, I say just sit me up in the corner and let me read everything I want to read until I can no longer read, then it will be time for me to go. I just completed an Advance Directive which clearly states what you want to have happen with yourself when you are no longer functional. If I turn into a bumbling idiot, I want someone to pull the plug. Please don't keep me alive just because.

How am I physically? This is simple. Things wear out. Those muscles and sinew and do-it-all-night capabilities have their time in the sun, but that is for competing for a mate, for a place in the world, for procreation, and to launch one's life. By about 45 or 50, one senses the inevitable state of cruising along as you are able, preserving as many body parts as possible. I exercise on a regular basis: cardio Monday, Wednesday, and Friday, yoga/core flexibility Tuesday, Thursday, and Saturday. I do this schedule starting at 6 am each morning. Sunday is my Day of Rest. Weekends, I always have some ongoing projects around the house, some gardening, and maintaining our vehicles. I deeply agree with the concept of Use It or Lose It.

I believe that for my age, I am in very good condition. I am physically able to do most everything I want or need to do, and I am in overall good health. But I've slowed down. Some things take a little longer, some take a lot longer, but I can still get it done. I do regret that some fixit and build it things I used to do myself, I now feel I have to hire someone else to do.

I have had two bouts with cancer. I was fortunate to discover the relatively invisible bladder cancer. It is not curable, but with monitoring, it is not lethal. I have been living with this cancer since 2016. Another fortunate break resulted from the bladder monitoring: my urologist noticed my PSA numbers going up and referred me to a specialist in prostate cancer. That cancer was detected early, and it was eradicated completely. I am forever indebted to my urologist for his decisive action. We have since become good friends.

Am I sexually active? Only in my mind. The prostate cancer treatment left me with Erectile Dysfunction. The Blue Pill is an option, but my wife and I have curtailed most sexual interludes over the past few years. Our affection for one another has become more cozy physical contact, holding hands, and kissing. Hey, who doesn't like kissing? We both enjoyed sexuality in earlier days, but now it is not so important. What is important is to be intimate, to do things together, to be there for each other. In short, to remain in love with each other. My wife is a wonderful person: strong, smart, generous, and genuine. After all the years I lived alone, it is much better to have a good partner whom you care for and cares for you. I learned that from my wife who I love very much. Make someone happy, make just one someone happy. Words to live by.

I don't use a cane or a walker, but I am partial to driving my sportscar on a twisty country road in the early morning sunshine. I have had a passion for cars and motorcycles all my life. I suppose that is foreign to many people, but there is a whole group of us out there who share that passion. An appreciation for some cars that are so special that many people gather around for rallies, for track days, for concours, for just getting together on Sunday mornings for Cars & Coffee. It's partly for an appreciation for the mechanical skill of some truly remarkable automobiles, the aesthetics of the design, the thrill of driving a car that performs at a level that is incredible. If you've never driven a car on a track at something close to the limits of the car's capability, it would be hard to understand the thrill of getting it right for an entire lap. Better than sex!

I have a similar relationship with motorcycles. When I was in high school, my best friend and I had motorcycles, and we rode them everywhere. We learned how to control them at speed and still stay alive. There is something about riding that is also foreign to many people who have not been on motorcycles. I understand that there is danger, but to ride, you begin to become more tuned into traffic around you. You see the drivers of cars who are not seeing you, who are distracted, who are on the phone, putting on makeup, or slapping the kids, and DON'T SEE YOU! You drive defensively, you anticipate and always plan for an escape route.

But the best times on a motorcycle are with other friends on motorcycles going for a ride in a place out in the open country where you can ride without a lot of people in cars, on the twisty bits and the high-speed sweepers when the motorcycle becomes part of you, an extension of your being. And that is a place that is truly existential.

In 2007, I was out for a motorcycle ride on my own in a cool morning in an area I have ridden many times before. It got warmer and I was thinking of a place to stop and remove some of my layers of clothing. I let my mind wander for just a few seconds and got into a turn carrying way too much speed. I could see that I was going to leave the road, but the bike was going too fast, and I dumped it, going ass over teakettle. That landed me in the hospital with a fractured rib, a lacerated spleen, and a broken collar bone.

I curtailed my riding for a time, but the urge was too great, and I started riding again, although with a much higher level of self-preservation. I limited my riding to outings with friends when we trailered the bikes to getaway places and rode as a group on a planned route with a chase vehicle. As much fun as that was, my riding was giving my wife a lot of heartache. Every time I went away on a ride it put my wife in tears. As much as I love to ride, I could not bear to see her so sad. I decided to give up the motorcycles and have not ridden since.

My mother is 105 years old. She is the sweetest, kindest, most loving mother imaginable. I spent much of my earlier life as a bachelor and during those years she was my best friend, my confidant, my cheerleader. Unfortunately, she is deep in dementia now and has lost much of her cognitive functioning, but she remains cheerful, always with a smile, unafraid and unaware of what day it is. I love her and I have no doubt that she loves me, when she finally figures out who I am.

My father was a good man, the most honest person I've known, but he was emotionally stunted. He had a difficult childhood, had to fend for himself at an early age. He never got past the 7th Grade, but he went to WW II as a soldier in the South Pacific, came home and started a family. He worked for the Post Office for 40 years, brought home the bacon, never strayed, got it done.

My father taught me how to use tools, to diagnose and fix things, to stick to it and get the job done. I know he loved me, but we did not interact on an emotional plane. My father always demanded the best of me and when I was younger, I didn't really get that. I thought he was just a hard ass, but later on, I got that he wanted me to give it my best shot, don't call it in, whatever it is. The tenderest time I had with my dad was when he retired, and I was in my undergraduate years. He was not a formally educated man and in his later years, we switched roles: he looked to me for guidance and for me to be the leader in our family after he had a series of strokes. Some of the best connections I had with him were in his last years. My father passed away in 1994.

I have one sister two years my senior. She provides primary care for our mother, and for that, I am truly grateful. She is retired and our mother lives with her.

My wife has children by a previous marriage, and they have children. I have some participation in their lives, a sort of uncle grandpa. The youngest is into cars and driving on track days, and we have bonded in this common interest.

Spiritually, I have no illusions regarding an afterlife. This is it. To all those people who plan on an extended engagement in Heaven, I say good luck with that, I hope it works out for you for all eternity, but for me, my only hope is that my ashes will be in the ocean and feeding some life form way beyond me. I'll be gone.

I have a good life, but I am very concerned about what is happening in our country right now. I never saw this coming, that factual reality would be overcome, denied in favor of lies, conspiracy theories, and the ravings of madmen, that fascism could win out over democracy, greed over brotherly love, that we might destroy the only place in the universe we can live.

I am very concerned to see that a faction of Christianity in this country seeks to impose their beliefs on the country, seeks a country that is governed by Christian Nationalists. I thought we learned the lesson of church and state separation, finally, but now that is in question. My only hope is that most people want peace, opportunity for all, justice of laws not of men, a commonwealth, not tribalism. I hope there are enough of us.

9

11-7-42

How do I feel emotionally? Scared, nervous, at times fortunate that I still feel useful. If I no longer feel useful, I want to be gone. Although most of the time I'm not ready to be gone, because I want to see our country recover from the horrible place, we are now in with such a polarized population. But I think it will take decades probably to get past where we now are…if we ever do! So, for this reason I feel quite depressed because I will obviously die not having any assurance that our democracy can survive and that my grandsons will grow up in a safe society. With more signs of racism, homophobia, antisemitism, I fear that we may experience what my parents did fleeing from Hitler.

And physically, so far, I'm OK. I'm on meds for blood pressure, for reflux, for a genetic tendency to get blood clots, for incontinence, and probably a few more things, but glad there are meds.

How do I feel about myself? As I started to say above, I feel fortunate that I am still useful to my community for my work on boards and in my blog/newsletter/action alert. People give me nice feedback saying they greatly appreciate the things I share.

Another area I have a lot of confusing feelings about is being useful as a caregiver. My husband could not live independently without my taking care of him. If I had a heart attack or stroke and died, our kids (very far way) would have to put him in a home for dependent seniors with memory challenges. But being a caregiver for someone with dementia and bipolarity is not easy or fun. I'm grateful that much of the time he is a happy, sweet person, and we're enjoying life together. We try to share as often as possible the things we feel grateful about, knowing that is much better than when we're irritable and defensive. The latter are the trying times.

As I said above, I'm ok physically. I'm able to walk each day for about 60–90 minutes with my husband depending on how strong we feel. We started that with the COVID pandemic. I'm basically a couch potato. Don't like exercise, but since I know that exercise is good for both of us, I make it a top priority. I usually don't miss a day unless it's raining (almost never happens) or I have an important conflict. My husband won't walk in the morning which is when I have more energy. I won't walk when it's over 70° and the sun is beating down. We have a nice path we walk around the neighborhood and we have found walls that we can sit on to rest about every 15 minutes or so.

We hold hands and people have stopped us to say they hope they will have a nice relationship to walk and hold hands when they get older. I have to tell them honestly; we're not holding hands because we're so romantic, we're holding hands so we won't fall down. He has had two falls where he broke a bone in his hand, which the orthopedist says is no big deal, but if you break a hip that is a BIG deal. So, I hold onto his hand fairly tightly and pull him up whenever he seems unstable and might go down.

The problem that worries me the most is something that has happened rarely, but I hate and is embarrassing. When we've been on our long walk, I've suddenly had to go to the bathroom and we are mostly 15- or 20-minutes' walk away from a park toilet or our house. In three years, I've had a poop accident twice, I'm guessing. The urge comes on suddenly and I can't hold it until I get home. I don't think anyone has known, and my husband wouldn't even know if I didn't tell him. But I absolutely hate it and the doctors I've told don't seem to have a cure for this. I try to go before we walk, but sometimes it doesn't help. The walking gets the digestive system moving. And then you have to go. Ugh! I only mention this embarrassing incontinence because I think it's always helpful to know that others might be having the same problem and might be too embarrassed to talk about it or even tell the doctor.

Concerning sexuality, we do not have sex. My husband was never very interested. So, the lack of sexual activity is not because we've gotten old, but because he was never very interested in sex. I occasionally have an orgasm with a vibrator.

About canes and walkers, I only used a walker when I had a hemangioma in my left hip and couldn't put much weight on my left side. It was helpful and I was very grateful that a friend went to the Loan Closet and picked one up for me. When we get older, it becomes necessary at times to have friends who help and sometimes we even have to ask, hard as that is.

I do have family. My daughter and her husband and two kids, 8 and 11 live on the east coast. She is very creative and bright, but is not so good at answering texts, emails, or calls. It makes me feel that she doesn't love me, but it might just be that she can't manage taking care of two kids with multiple challenges. Our son lives in the Northwest. He is single and is also living with a lot of stress, but most of his life he's been good about keeping in touch. He calls us a couple of times a month. He is a worry for us too. He is 55, and single. And happily, both of our kids are as politically progressive as we are. So, we don't have a polarized family that can't talk to each other. We enjoy talking and strongly support each other's work and beliefs, although at times there is stress between our two kids. We hope to get some family therapy to help with that.

In my earlier years I was always politically active, always did teaching, training, and counseling. It was VERY worthwhile, very gratifying. I miss the interaction and knowing I'm helping others, but I still manage to be supportive of people even now that I'm not teaching or counseling.

I retired from teaching college courses at age 73, when I felt my husband needed more caregiving and when I was starting to have trouble thinking of the words I wanted. I was proud that my student evaluations were very high and I wanted to go out with them high and not wait till students would say, she can't remember our names or remember the words she wants. And yes, I was good at what I did. I was proud that when I had 90 students each semester, I usually had learned all of their names by the second or third week of the semester. And students told me they were amazed that I knew them so quickly and liked that I knew who they were.

I was also proud that students often told me that my class was their favorite college class. So, I definitely miss that nice feedback. I miss teaching a little, but I've kept quite busy so I have other things that make me feel I'm doing something helpful. I've tried to be supportive of friends who have lost their partners or had to deal with illness.

I NEVER made enough money to support myself. Luckily my husband was a full-time tenured professor. I worked for a nonprofit organization for 20 years and I made half as much as my husband.

I didn't have a graduate degree and wished I had one, but was afraid of going to grad school because reading had always been hard for me, and the university which offered a Masters in Social Work was a 4-hour drive from our home. I was scared to even apply because only one out of ten applicants to the MSW program were accepted. In talking to one of the faculty there I told her that I'd have to go part time because I didn't want to lose my job. Then I said, *"Oh gees, I'm 52 years old. Forget it. I won't get through till I'm 56 years old."*

She said, *"Dear, I hate to tell you this, but you'll be 56 years old anyway! Do you want to be 56 years old with a Masters degree or 56 years old without one?"*

That changed my mind. And I applied and got in. For four years I drove four hours to the university every Tuesday night, stayed overnight so I could be in class at 8am on Wednesday, and at noon drove back home. In four years, I had an MSW and then two universities called me and asked me to teach as an adjunct. I loved teaching at the University and then in retirement at City College.

Financially now, I worry about how long our savings will last. Fortunately, my parents left me a nice inheritance, without which we wouldn't have been able to buy our house in 2002. If we don't need to hire caregivers, or go into a nursing home, I think we'll manage well financially. But you never know. I want so much to leave our two kids the same kind of inheritance that my parents left me. So, I hope we won't need expensive care. Neither of our kids could take care of us financially. Neither has the job security that my husband's job gave him.

Considering religious beliefs, I'm a devout atheist. I don't believe in life after death. We have donated our bodies to UCLA Med Center, as my parents also did. I feel very good about that. I like helping science and like saving the money of cremation for my kids.

I developed a new interest in retirement, that of photographer. People had often told me I took good pictures and captured the excitement or spirit of events that I covered. I became the amateur photographer for political events, marches, protests that I loved and wanted to document. Thanks to a dear friend, I was coached on how to use a new camera. As an old lady I found it hard to learn so much of what the camera could do, but as long as I could take nice closeup photos of faces and their wonderful expressions, my photos were appreciated by most of my subjects.

The skill at capturing the best of people in my photos, helped me with another thing I've enjoyed doing in my old age. I've made six books celebrating an older person's life with many photos and statements collected from their family and friends telling what they appreciate, admire and love about the honored person. It is a job which takes hours and hours for sometimes a year, but I so strongly believe that we should say all the nice things about people while they can enjoy them, not after they die. I made one of these books for my husband's 80th birthday, another for my brother-in-law's 90th birthday, another for our first Mayor's 90th Birthday, another for my college roommate's dying husband, and one for my dear friend's retirement from teaching Social Work, the one who told me I'd be 56 anyway. The sixth one was for a younger recipient, my daughter's 50th Birthday.

10

10-26-47

Aging is an unexpected challenge. Between creaky knees, shoulders that "catch" emanating pain and discomfort, and occasional hemorrhoids, I feel GREAT! Emotionally I've never been better: I have accomplished so much in my 74 years and have fewer and fewer needs. I no longer have to prove myself, answer to anyone, bow to a higher earthly being, or search for excitement. I no longer have to be someone I'm not. I've been there, done that. My adult years have been marked with incredible luck and fortune (mostly non-monetary). My heart is full of gratitude for having what I have.

As mentioned, I'm not in the best physical condition, but not handicapped yet. I'm overweight, which causes me strife and regret. My wardrobe is filled with clothes that cover the unwanted bulges. As a result, I have high blood pressure and am pre-diabetic. Arthritis (a family curse) is creeping into the joints, but I'm determined to keep active. My skin sags and is marked by scars from injuries, surgeries, skin cancer procedures, and old bug bites. I am however flattered when people say, "I can't believe you are 70+."

Am I sexually active? This depends on how you define sexually active. Even though we haven't had intercourse in several years, we (my husband and I) still can't keep our hands off each other…does that count? We make out almost every morning and groping is big in my household. Must I continue?

I do not use a cane…knock on wood.

My family provides a strong foundation for my well-being. I have 4 siblings (including a twin brother) that I adore and cherish. I am a big part of their families as well. They have always given me strength, support and unconditional love.

My husband of 38 years is my rock and I wake each day feeling blessed and grateful. Though we have our moments, we always feel secure in the relationship which is steady and enduring.

My husband has a son from a former marriage who married and has produced 3 granddaughters.

I am fortunate to get grandkids without having reared any children. Being a "step grandmother" has its challenges and I have learned to step back and keep my mouth shut.

After earning a Master's degree in Public Health, I have been in various health education positions in 4 different public health departments in California. My career ended as the Executive Director of the American Lung Association. Worthwhile? ABSOLUTELY. The work fits in with my political leanings which embraces the well-being of the whole of the population. Community Health allowed me to find compassion for those of different races, genders, sexual orientation, ethnicities and languages. I was good at community organizing and bringing people together for a common cause. I don't miss the bureaucracies, but I miss the work, the other professionals with whom I worked, and the comradery I felt with my coworkers and those I met on the job. And I made enough money to assure my independence and live comfortably.

Now I am financially set because of my husband's and my pensions. Plus, I inherited money from my family that allows for non-essential expenses, especially travel.

Regarding spirituality, I do believe. I'm not sure what I believe, but I know there is a higher being/force. I'm not even sure there is a life after death, but I believe there is, and I'm not afraid to explore that realm.

Life has been good to me: I've been able to take advantage of many opportunities such as living and studying abroad (Sweden, Germany, Venezuela, Puerto Rico). I lived in Europe for two years, and two years in South America in the Peace Corps. Travel is a passion and I feel most fulfilled while discovering new lands. My values have not changed with age. My political interests reflect my values and with retirement, I have been able to politically advocate freely. Life is GOOD.

11

12-14-51

I feel pretty good emotionally, except that COVID has left me with many questions, and with some amount of fear for the future. It's similar to fears about the future for our children and grandchildren regarding climate change. The earth may kick us all off the planet one way or another in order to sustain itself. I'm shocked and sad that everyone does not understand this situation that we humans have put ourselves in. Time already has, or will soon run out on us, and we are not collectively taking on the responsibility to make the necessary changes to reverse our own destruction and the destruction of many other living things.

Physically? I'm in pretty good condition—working out most days and taking my regimen of vitamins and minerals. Getting good sleep most of the time. I feel pretty good physically!

And about myself? I don't have many good friends, and sometimes I wonder if I was so busy doing things (running a business, etc.) that I missed some things along the way. And, I don't think there's a way to go back in order to change things or make up for this lost time. That's the other thing, nothing stops the march of time.

My wife and I are happy to continue to be sexually active. About once a week does it for us.

Fortunately, there are no walking aids like a cane or a walker needed—YET!

I live with my wife. I have three children, all who live far away from us—I often wonder why that is, and what I may have done to make where we live unappealing to all three of them. I doubt they will ever come back to NEOH to live. Also, let's face it, the pandemic, which will still be with us for quite some time, has changed everything and most everyone. We have four grandchildren, all wonderful.

I founded and operated my own business for more than 40 years. I think it was very worthwhile, and I worked with many fine people and made some good relationships along the way. At the same time, I was a good provider for my family, and I was able to save enough for retirement. There are many days that I miss working when I owned my own company. After I sold it, the new owners were difficult for me to work with.

I was good at what I did. More than 50% of the time I made good decisions. I knew my clients and team members very well, and always tried to do the right thing—continuous improvements over time. And, yes, I made enough money as I said above. Enough to retire comfortably and do what I choose to do.

Spirituality and or religion and a life after death? Do I believe? Good question! Still working that out. I was raised Catholic, was an altar boy, left the church, came back when married with kids, left again after divorce, and am not happy with the Christian Church. My unhappiness with the Christian church comes from the hypocrisy that I observe and the exclusionary practices that I witness from time to time, which are very much not the teachings of Christ.

I do not believe in life after death, and feel that right now, this life is our chance and when it's over, it's over. I do believe in a lasting spiritual presence in the universe that will live on without me, mostly through the lives of those who are left behind.

It is strange to continue to grow older, because at some point one realizes that we will all reach an inevitable end, and now it's much closer than when we were in our younger years. And, there's no turning back, yet I still do not feel like I'm 70. Instead, I feel much younger. I am a scientist at heart, and I know that even this universe that we currently inhabit will come to an end someday, or maybe better put, it will change into something we cannot even imagine.

12

8-19-40

This morning I am very sad, lonely, and depressed because my sister and best friend is gone from this earth. I am also happy, because I told her how much I love her, not once but many times. I am physically unwell and am in treatment for lung and brain cancer and because I have little or no immune system, I suffer from joint and muscle pain. However, once I am on my feet in the morning, I get going. FATIGUE is my greatest enemy and I sit down often.

I feel pretty good about myself as I continue to do my volunteer work at my church (visiting shut-ins) and at a major hospital cuddling infants in the NICU. I am also friend, P.O.A and Executor for an elderly friend who has absolutely no family left. She is in a nursing home and is 94 years of age. My attitude is very positive because of my faith. My oncologists say that my positive attitude is very beneficial to my condition.

We are no longer sexually active.

I do not use a cane or walker but it is coming soon because at times I am quite wobbly. I wish I had my sister's black cane with the sparkly knob. I think I'll get myself one. She didn't use it, but often carried it in her basket. She said it made her feel chic. We laughed at that a lot.

I have a husband who is a great help to me, two sons and one daughter. We have one grandson aged 26 and two little girls 8 and 5. They are a great joy to me.

I worked the last 13 years of my working life for a Reinsurance firm. I don't miss going out to work but I certainly do miss my colleagues who were also my friends. As I was the eldest in the branch, I was also the Mother Hen. I was very good at my job in the accounting dept. and was recognized by the execs.

Financially we are very comfortable.

Spiritually I am at the top of my game and I surrender myself to God every single day saying, "Thy will be done."

No questions about technology? My friend suggested that I include that in my contribution because technology is such a mainstream issue these days. Some elders (her word for olders, she likes elders better) may have trouble keeping up. But, I'm good with it. I have a smart phone, an iPad, and a Kobo Reader. I text and I email. I shop on line. I bank on line, I email transfer. I use medical apps as available such as "My Chart" for appointments and test results. We have a Wi-Fi, streaming apps, and a pvr.

13

10-29-36

Emotionally I am fine. Sometimes there is loneliness but I enjoy watching sport programs and have family support. I have two step children and one daughter. There are four grandchildren and most live in Southern California near me.

Physically I have a bad back and have had two shoulder surgeries. General health is good for an 85-year-old but I also have some hearing problems.

I am happy with my life and there is no sexual activity.

I use a walking stick for balance and steadiness.

I live alone and have some female friends whom I go to dinner with occasionally.

I worked for the water company in San Dimas for 40 years managing field operations in the San

Dimas and Claremont areas. Loved my work and was involved in many civic activities such as rotary and San Dimas Chamber of Commerce. I am a past president of the Chamber and chaired the annual City BBQ for 25 years. Very rewarding. I retired at 62 because my wife was ill.

I made good investments on stocks, especially Tesla, so it those have given me a secure future. Finances are no problem.

I am a believer but not an active church attendee. I feel I am spiritual and believe in God. I think there is a life ever after. If I come back, I want to come back as a rooster in Hawaii and have a lot of chicks.

(This was dictated to a second party for our use here.)

14

11-4-36

Emotionally I am pretty stable. My days are spent working in my profession and after hours involved with family and civic activities.

I miss my husband everyday as he was very special. He was my second husband but the man of my dreams. Not a day went by that he did not tell me he loved me. Even though I am busy there are still some lonely times and tears. It has been almost 9 years since his passing. Due to the happiness I had, I wanted a friend to share my later years.

After 62 years I reconnected with an old high school boyfriend. He has filled a void in my life. I was having dinner with friends and we were reminiscing and the husband had gone to high school with my friend. I contacted him by letter and he called me back and that was the start of a lovely friendship and sharing a lot of hugs. He had never married so I filled a missing link in his life. The three of us drove to the beach to meet for the first time in 62 years and had a wonderful time. We then went sailing several weeks later. Since then, the two of us have traveled several times across country with other smaller trips. We are involved in each other's family occasions. We laugh as we say we have a triangle to visit, he living at the beach, and my homes in the flatlands and desert.

Physically I can't do all I would like as my knees are bad and should be replaced, but I have been listed as a medium risk for surgery so I would rather endure the pain and be alive than take a chance on surgery, since I have lost several friends after this type of surgery. I still walk on my own but once in a while when I am out with my daughter and we have a distance to walk I will use the walker.

I have been in my insurance profession for over 53 years as I still enjoy it but the time is coming in the near future when it is time to retire and sell my business. I am also managing a 21 unit office building that my husband left me, so both take up a lot of time. It is getting time to sell that as well. I enjoy my involvement in clubs and city activities, but a lot of friends are passing so I find I am one of the oldest members.

I have five daughters who are very attentive to me for which I am very blessed. Eight grandchildren plus one who passed away, four great grandchildren and one great, great grandson who is eight weeks old and a beautiful baby. We are a very close-knit family and do a lot together which is wonderful.

I know my body is getting old and I feel all the aches and pains but mentally, thank God I have all my senses. I keep getting comments from friends who say, "You are still working." I respond, yes, because I like what I do and like being busy.

I am fortunate to have had a good life, there have been some major/minor glitches along the way but that is life and we go on.

I do believe in God and pray each day. When the children were growing, we went to church every Sunday but since they have left home, I don't attend church regularly but try to live a Christian life.

Financially I am able to live comfortably.

15

4-7-50

Ten or so years ago, it dawned on me that time was marching on despite my denial and resistance to the notion that I would EVER become an "Older," a senior citizen and/or an elderly person. Unfortunately, here I am, and now I feel the best way to deal with it is recognition (or at least partial recognition).

Every day I take a moment to stand back and be grateful as a way to remind me that I am essentially in good shape. That leads me to my belief in positive thinking, which definitely helps me maintain a reasonably good emotional and physical state. Of course, there are certain joints and some "bodily functions" that have deteriorated over time, but for the most part all is good. However, I am frustrated by the microscopic print on labels and other items which are difficult, if not impossible, to read without excellent light and a magnifying glass.

When I was younger, I thought I'd get over my vanity of wanting to be taller and thinner, but, alas, that hasn't happened. I keep trying to lose those pounds I gained since retiring in 2014, but that probably is not going to happen, not to mention I've lost more than a ½ inch in height, which brings me down to an even 5-foot-tall human being. Oh, well.

Enjoying (for the most part) a 50-year plus marriage has been more than a stroke of luck in my life, both mentally and physically. We are still close in all ways and our communication skills have gotten much, much better over time.

We have a very small family (two children), with no prospects for grandchildren, which was one of my expectations. Of course, it wasn't my choice to make, so I honor their decisions. Most importantly, our children are caring and smart adults of which I am very proud. I do have to admit, however, over the last several years, they have been slowly, and with finesse, checking in on their parents more than they used to. I did the same thing as my parents aged, so I guess I can't complain.

I was lucky to work alongside my husband for several years in the broadcasting industry. We learned a lot about one another during that time and, even more importantly, learned about each other's strengths and limitations. After about 10 years, I made a change into the non-profit arena, having many opportunities to launch new or build on existing programs. I think I was pretty good at it, and I was fortunate to be well paid, which has made retirement much easier. Fortunately, our financial situation is stable providing us with enough money for periodic travel and no worries about day-to-day needs.

Let me turn again to my husband. In mid-2019, he was diagnosed with Parkinson's Disease (PD). While we both knew something was "off," we never would have guessed that it would be something we (both) would live with for the rest of our marriage. From the age of 12, my husband loved and played music, and when he retired in 2013, his retirement goals were to travel and, most of all, to get back into his music. He approached his music with gusto. Of course, one of the first thoughts he had after diagnosis was how would he continue following his musical mistress (my label not his). Despite PD, he's worked hard to maintain his voice, hand dexterity and overall movement with various physical therapies and many, many daily dog walks with me and our dog, Jasper.

One irony has been that exercise was never something he enthusiastically pursued, but now it's exercise that is keeping his Parkinson's progression somewhat at bay. A frustrating challenge for both of us is not knowing how PD will affect him one day to the next. Is today's fatigue, for example, due to overall aging or PD? Because PD progresses differently in each person, his future is unpredictable with respect to where PD may take him next year or in 5 to 10 years. However, we have been proactive and positive by educating ourselves and accessing appropriate physicians and support services to fight back vigorously at a chronic disease that has no clear or foreseeable timetable or path.

As I indicated before, I believe positivity is one of the most important aspects of a healthy, happy life. I don't consider myself a religious person, but I do believe there is something greater than I. That perspective has helped me get through various challenges I've encountered in my life.

Recently I was searching through some old boxes from my parents (and grandparents), and I found a small page from "This Week Magazine." Evidently it was published in *Reader's Digest* in 1945. The article is titled "How to Stay Young." The piece was based on the poem, "Youth," written by Samuel Ullman around 1918. It hung over General MacArthur's desk at his Manila Headquarters. I thought I'd share some excerpts with you.

> *"Youth is not a time of life—it is a state of mind; it is a temper of the will, a quality of the imagination, a vigor of the emotions, a predominance of courage over timidity, of the appetite for adventure over love of ease.*
>
> *Nobody grows old by merely living a number of years; people grow old only by deserting their ideals. Years wrinkle the skin, but to give up enthusiasm wrinkles the soul.*
>
> *You are as young as your faith, as old as your doubt; as young as your self-confidence, as old as your fear, as young as your hope, as old as your despair."*

Need I say more?

16

10-24-46

I was born on October 24, 1946, the same date that the United Nations was formed in the following year. This statement is my personal narrative about getting older, not about being old. Rather than the terms *old* and *older*, I prefer the concept of *elder*. Elder to me embodies a conscious choice to play a specific role in society in which I draw from my experiences to serve others.

Having said that I suppose I should discuss how I feel emotionally. I have tended to be a late bloomer in the various aspects of my life, and I think I have taken a long time to mature emotionally. However, I have vibrant emotions. I have a lot of passion. I love being surrounded by art and beauty, love to wear stylish clothes, and adore being in the company of good friends.

Physical health has always been important to me and I have made huge efforts over the course of my lifetime to stay physically fit. I began studying dance very seriously at age 23 and underwent strenuous training in ballet, modern dance, and jazz. Over the course of years I performed in dance companies in Los Angeles and Santa Barbara. I have also taught dance in formal studio settings and currently conduct gentle stretching sessions with patients at Santa Barbara Cottage Hospital in their department of Psychology and Addiction Medicine.

I swim usually twice a week and maintain a personal stretching regimen at home. The payoff is that I can still move about gracefully and rise to a standing position from the floor without assistance.

I was diagnosed with prostate cancer in 2012 and also have glaucoma, but the cancer was caught in time and there has not been a recurrence. I have been treated for glaucoma for years by a wonderful ophthalmologist and my condition has been stable for a number of years. I am dealing with an old ankle injury that never healed properly and am currently in physical therapy for that. Overall, however, I would say that I am in excellent health.

Nothing would make me happier than to meet a wonderful man that I could partner with. I have a lot of interest in sex although I am only occasionally sexually active. The infrequency of sexual activity is not necessarily an outcome of getting older. Although I was more sexually active as a younger man there were always long periods of inactivity. I think that part of this was due to my discomfort with my own sexuality.

As a teenager in the Midwest in the 1960s I never had much discussion with my family about sexual matters. There was no one in my environment that I felt I could talk to about my emerging sexual identity. So, I tended to avoid that aspect of my life and focused instead on artistic achievement. The treatments I received for prostate cancer included the implantation of radioactive seeds directly into my prostate. They eliminated the cancer but also damaged many of the nerves that stimulate an erection. So now I have much exploration to do to discover new modes to sexual satisfaction.

Once I left home in my 20s, I lived with a succession of roommates for a number of years. I have lived alone in my current apartment for the last 30 years. I never married or had children. I do experience loneliness, but often felt lonely as a young man as well. I do participate in a group called Lavender Elders that is sponsored by Pacific Pride Foundation here in Santa Barbara. That group has been a meaningful source of social support.

So, all things considered I feel proud of my achievements. I studied hard during my youth and avoided drugs and alcohol. I earned a PhD in Theatre Arts from UCSB in 2005, taught for 28 years in the Theatre Arts Department at Santa Barbara City College, and have a post retirement position at Cottage Hospital. In March 2022 I also wrote and performed a one-person play about my life's journey titled *The War Shirt* that can be viewed online at luketheatre.org. These are achievements that I am very proud of, and I feel a great sense of satisfaction that I have never wasted my life.

I never made lots of money although I always worked very hard. I tended to value artistic achievement over making money. I do receive a small pension from Santa Barbara City College and a small allotment from Social Security. My current position at Cottage Hospital has really helped to ease financial stress. I am currently generating $70,000 a year, but in today's world that does not go all that far and I always need to be careful about managing my financial resources. I am also repaying a student loan that financed my graduate studies.

In 1974 I was age 27 and living in Los Angeles. At that time, I was introduced to the practice of Nichiren Buddhism. I became a member of the organization that is now known as Soka Gakkai International of the USA (SGI-USA) *Soka Gakkai* translates from the Japanese language as "value creating society" and refers to the human capacity to create something of value from all adverse circumstances.

This particular Buddhist practice has been a radical departure from the much more fundamentalist Baptist worldview that I was raised with. Nichiren Buddhism apprehends a fundamental law of life that expresses itself as both life and death. Therefore, this law is ever present in its innumerable physical manifestations as well as in its latent state that we identify as death. Buddhism views death itself as an intermediary condition that will give rise once again to a manifest form of life. I draw much inspiration and comfort from this concept.

In conclusion I would like to say that I view myself as a work in progress. I am a dancer, a performer, a theatre practitioner, a healer, and a teacher. My tasks and challenges now are to bring all of these abilities together in a new and original synthesis—a final statement perhaps about the significance of my present lifetime in this world!

17

7-8-47

I feel good emotionally and comfortable in my own skin. My body feels worn and tired. Not able to walk as far or do steps like before. My energy is much less and the desire to do some things has waned. But I feel comfortable with who I am and I don't worry about what others think of me as long as I am not hurting others.

We need to be ourselves and our own best friend. I've learned to not be too hard on myself when I make mistakes, as that's how we can learn.

I'm usually "the glass is 1/2 full" person.

I am not physically fit—continually need to work on this and I do enjoy strenuous gardening and dancing. That said, my 76-year-old retired husband and I had a bout with Covid and I tell you about all that below.

My latest drama was my "moderate" heart murmur advanced to "severe." Fortunately, I was able to get my valve replacement through the femoral artery. It's called TAVR. It's a 45-minute surgery done while you are awake and talking. You have anesthesia, and feel no pain. You do not need to be on any blood thinner except baby aspirin. I am doing heart rehab once a week.

My hip decided to go South on me, so am doing rehab two times a week. Also, just healed from ear-crystal vertigo. I've got a new "Game Plan." I have a set rehab outfit…jogging pants, and an EKG—loose tee shirt. I also, have one outfit designated for Dr. appts.

Makes Life a Snap!

My husband and I have no sexual activity anymore.

I do not use a cane or walker—but have while recovering from injuries or surgeries. It was an adjustment, but workable.

We have two adult children and four grandchildren. I live with my husband of 53 years.

I worked for the Telephone Co., then was a customer service rep for the Gas Co. prior to marriage.

Then, opted to be a stay-at-home mom while raising children…my most important and rewarding job!! My job, as I've said, as a stay-at-home mom was extremely worthwhile and I'm proud to have raised two caring and amazing adults.

I wasn't into making lots of money, but enough to live and pay bills and a bit of savings.

I do not miss working outside the home.

No, financial considerations are not an issue. Our financial situation is fine.

And now my Covid story. Covid hits older folk with a punch! We did not get vaccinated because of some of the things I read but we wore masks and never knew how we got it. But got it we did in January of this year (2022). I was extremely weak—could only walk from bed to bathroom to recliner. My husband caught it soon thereafter. He mostly slept and barely ate. And things went downhill.

Concerned about my husband's decline, I called 911. He had to wait outside in a chair. They checked his vitals and decided he did not need to be hospitalized and we went home.

In a couple days, things worsened. He was even chewing his daily meds instead of swallowing! I called 911. They, again, thought vitals were passable. He correctly answered three simple questions they asked him. They said they would take him to the hospital only if I insisted. I insisted.

Our kids were keeping the phone lines busy checking on us during the day and wanting to come help. Thinking I could handle it ok I had been saying no since they both live a distance.

A few hours later, the hospital called and said, you can come and get him now. They gave him home rest for Covid. I quickly called our son, who lives three hours away to come help. I was weak and not physically able to drive over to pick my husband up and did not want any of our friends to be exposed. So, I asked the hospital if they could call a taxi since they had no other game plan. They would call me back and let me know, because I wanted to be sitting by the window to wait for his arrival.

No call. Then the front door burst open and my husband "ran" into the house yelling, "I need money!!"

I almost fainted. I grabbed money and a generous tip and actually made it out to pay the driver. My husband followed me. He was on high anxiety adrenaline. Time for naps.

Our Son came bearing KFC! The Cavalry had arrived! He was fully masked and kept a hefty distance. He gave us full service and security. He remained until the next day when our daughter flew in to save the day! She was outfitted in battery-powered fan bionic headgear for safety.

She shopped, cooked, bought and assembled handicap devices, cleaned, laundered, helped with bill paying and pills. She stayed with us for almost three weeks and was a life-saver!

My husband was deteriorating mentally and physically. One evening we took all his vitals. Oxygen was 88 and 90, not good. The next morning, I went into his room and he had three pair of underwear and socks on. We again called 911.

Again, they were not thinking he was in trouble. His oxygen was maybe 92 and he answered a couple questions ok. We said, ask more. They asked what year it was and who the President was—he failed. He was hospitalized for six days—on oxygen, prednisone, and insulin. His brain fog was horrible. He told us, while talking on the phone from the hospital, that he was out of clean underwear, so was washing some out on the floor of his shower! He is a very clean man…

He is doing very well now—his brain fog has lifted and he's 98%! We are Thankful!! We are doing as well as can be expected.

As far as believing goes, I am a Christian and believe in Jesus Christ as my Lord and Savior. Jesus resides in every heart. We need to admit we have sinned and accept Jesus and will have ever-lasting life. As I said, Jesus resides in every heart. That's the spiritual nudge you feel when doing right or wrong…your "gut" feeling. I have no fear of dying because Jesus is always with me and gives eternal life.

Things To Help With Aging:
You Need a Huge Sense of Humor.
Never Expect Life to be a Plan A, prepare for Plan B or C.
Stock up on Sympathy Cards…saves many trips to the store.
Getting Botox for frown lines makes me feel more cheerful while watching skin sag and wither.
Realize everyone's dealing with their own stuff—you're not being "picked on."
I'm never lonely—sometimes overwhelmed with too much going on.
We are close, by telephone, with our kids on a regular basis. They are our Joy!

My fun in life is going out and singing karaoke, dancing to live bands, and game nights with friends. Find the Joy in life!

Immerse yourself into nature, as that is a lifesaver!

18

11-5-38

Emotionally I feel pretty good. I'm basically a happy go lucky kind of guy. I try not to let things bother me or get in my way. But I have a tendency to over think things and that does interfere with the emotions. I think that's because I am fairly sensitive. So that causes the over thinking part. Other than that, I am very happy with my life. And that is because I keep myself busy. I am not happy if I don't have something to do. I am landscaping the new house I bought here in Arizona about three years ago and I build things out of wood. Tables, fences, planter boxes and so forth.

Generally, I feel fine. I feel good. I am happy with my physical condition. Not many aches and pains. The right knee has some arthritis beginning to show up and my left index figure is crooked and difficult to use. But we learn how to do things out of necessity. I'm able to get around very well and take care of myself. I am thankful for that. I'm very lucky. I am a little slower than I used to be and sore muscles show up more often than in the past. But that is to be expected so I don't let it bother me. One thing that does aggravate me though is sometimes when I reach for something or attempt to put the salt container back on the shelf, I miss the mark by a fraction of an inch and oops, something gets spilled or knocked over. Hand eye coordination? And that is very annoying. My motto is "Deal with it." I'll have it engraved on my headstone above my grave. So, no complaints here.

I've had a couple of operations, right shoulder rotator cup replacement, a tumor on my right Adrenal gland removed (Pheochromocytoma), along with a Carotid endarterectomy on my right carotid where they removed excess plaque. I wear hearing aids and have had two procedures on my left ear. That has improved the hearing there and they tell me it will get substantially better. We'll see. I have corneal dystopia, which causes a double vision. As a result, I use saline eye drops to help with that. Works fairly well. Like I said, deal with it.

I live alone and have for 35 years. I have a degree in Math and a Masters in Systems Engineering. I spent my early career days working in the Space Exploration area and then moved on to the Defense area working on the F-14A aircraft as a weapons systems analyst and then as a Flight Test Engineer. That last part was the best part of my career. That was just FUN.

I was raised in a medical family. My father was an MD, Family Practice. He delivered all of my friends and schoolmates. Our upbringing was one where you did your work before you went out to play. And if you whined because you were bored, you were told to go play with your toys or go out and hoe the weeds in the rose garden. The rule was discipline and if you were bad and got into trouble, you got a spanking.

But that doesn't mean that it wasn't a happy childhood growing up. We played outside and rode our bicycles where ever we wanted to. Even down to Puddingstone reservoir, which was several miles away. Kick the can. Hide and seek. Let's build a fort using the bales of hay that Ole Mr. Shaffer just left behind in the field next door. Let's go fishing. Chief Case wants me to shoot some of the pigeons in his palm trees in front of his house, with my 22-air gun. We played baseball and football in the park kitty corner from our house. We also climbed up the trees there to look into the bird nests to see the baby birds. Yes, life was good.

After high school I joined the Navy for a couple of years and then went to college to get my math degree. What followed was a period of four marriages and divorces. That was from 1961 to 1992. By that time, I had left my chosen career path and ventured into some other activities. I built three houses with my last ex-wife and then moved to Colorado solo. I lived in the high Rocky Mountains at about the 9,500-foot level in a cabin I bought there. I loved living there. I raised chickens and had quite a few experiences with the wildlife there while trying to protect my flocks. Bears, mountain lions, coyotes, bobcats, weasels and foxes. It took a while but I learned how to deal with the predators.

When I turned 80, after 22 years there, I decided that I had had enough of shoveling snow and decided to move to Arizona. I did that all by myself. Packed everything, took it to storage and hired a truck to move my stuff to my new home in Arizona. I'm pretty proud of that feat.

So here I am living a good life in my chosen location. I am very happy.

I am in very good physical shape for a guy my age. And for that I am very thankful. If I wasn't, I'm sure I wouldn't be as happy as I am. I take a few prescription drugs and some supplements. But nothing that if I stopped taking them would cause me to die. I pay attention to my physical wellness and if something new pops up I go online and research possible causes and cures. I also have good medical care which is a big plus.

I'm not an exercise freak but the amount of physical activity involved with landscaping and wood working causes a lot of sweating, especially when it's hot. I love how I feel after a day of digging holes for bushes or bending and leaning while working with wood. I also walk our dog. (She belongs to my best friend and I take care of her during weekdays while she works. I've been doing that since she was a pup. We call her "our" dog.) I also lift weights to keep my arms in shape and also do knee bends and stretches once in a while. I do not use/need a cane nor a walker.

I eat healthily. Meat, potatoes and veggies. That's what they say is a well-rounded diet. Oatmeal in the morning, poached eggs at 10am or so, then lunch at 11, Then bananas, hard boiled eggs and an oatmeal cookie somewhere between 2 and 4pm. Dinner at 7 pm after a couple of scotch and sodas while watching a Western movie, which is my favorite part of the day.

It's been a long time since I've had any sex. That is basically my choice, as I have lived alone for a long time and don't really want to have a "girlfriend" as it would interfere with my (selfish?) current solo living arrangements. I don't get lonely. I have had girlfriends in the past, last one was sometime around 2005.

I have two female friends who I have known for 20 some years and we are very close. But no sexual activities. They are in their 50s so you can understand that. One of them lives in Colorado, where I met her 15 or so years ago. When I lived there, we would frequently go out to dinner. The other, whom I also met in Colorado, I've known for over 20 years and she followed me to Arizona after my move. She has established her own place and has a boyfriend in Colorado. We are dedicated to each other and are each other's helpmates. We're helping each other thru life. She is the owner of the dog I mentioned earlier. It's a great relationship and works out well for both of us. So, I am happy with my situation.

I have four siblings, two sisters, 86 and 80, and two brothers, 70 and 65. I have two daughters and four grandchildren. I also have nine great grandchildren. As stated earlier, I live alone. One daughter and her mother live nearby here in Arizona. The mother was my second wife and we have, after 50 years, reconnected. Her husband died last year. She and our daughter left California and moved here to Arizona. We have since picked up the relationship and are in contact on a regular basis. Not getting back together, just remaining friends. Our grandson also lives here in Arizona. It's family.

My other daughter lives in Washington State along with my three grandchildren and nine great grandchildren. I visit them at least once a year and we do "Zoom" sessions now and then. Great grandchildren are an interesting stimulation. Watching your progeny grow up is fascinating.

I was an engineer for most of my adult life. During my engineering career I worked in SoCal, Pascagoula, Mississippi, and Washington DC. In a way, I do miss working. I sometimes day dream about my old company calling me back to do more work in flight test on some new airplane. I read Aviation News and Space Technology to keep up on what's going on in the industry. But it is so nice to be able to wake up in the morning and do what you want to do that day, on your own schedule. I usually plan the day the night before as I fall asleep. I don't like interruptions, like going to the dentist or for some doctor appointment.

I don't particularly like to travel. I love working around my house and reading emails and catching up on what's going on in the world and in the tech area. I love new technology and the various new capabilities that are being produced. I consider what I'm doing to and for this house I moved into three years ago as my job. That's my work. And my joy.

I worked hard and did what was requested of me and I prospered. So, I guess by that standard I was good at what I did. I tried to do the best I could. I am dyslectic so I had to work a little bit harder to get it right. When I was living at home, back in the day, sometimes when I would slack off some, I remember my mom saying, "You're not living up to your potential." That thought always kept pushing me. (Oh, the virtue signaling. Lol.)

I wasn't rich, but I made enough money to always be able to buy my own house. And have the necessities of life. And a few luxuries like a sail boat. Early on, starting out, money was tight and there was never enough. During my first marriage I was going to college and working at night as a janitor. I put myself thru college, with some help from my parents. And during that period, I was poor. But working for the main goal made it OK. We got by.

Later in my career, the money situation got much better and we were good. Sometimes we over spent, though, and that got us into trouble. I finally figured out how to control and live under a budget. Credit cards are a good thing, but they can also lead to big trouble. That's a lesson I think a lot of people have a problem learning. All in all, we survived.

I am financially secure. I live comfortably and have what I need. Could always use more money, but that's always true with just about everybody, I think. If I had more, I would just put it into savings so how much is enough or too much. I'm happy with my income. Not worried because my monthly income is guaranteed. And there are savings and dividend paying stocks I own.

I was brought up in the Methodist church and baptized in 1948. So, I am Christian. I don't go to church, but I pray each night at about 2 am. Weird, huh. But to each his own. Believing in a God is based on Faith. I believe there is a higher being, like a God. When you look at nature and study the laws of physics, you see the order and you just know that there is something unique going on. Plants and trees have a vascular system called Xylem and Phloem, which transport nutrients and food between the roots and the leaves and other parts of the plants. We humans have our circulatory system that courses blood thru our bodies, performing similar functions. How did this happen? Not by accident I would suggest. So, we wonder if there is a God that did all this and when we can't answer these questions, we become the faithful, believing in a high order. Some call it God. One of the most interesting books I have read is "The Source," by James Michener. It is a study of the major religions and its conclusion is that there is just one God. Worshiped by all religions.

I have had a few strange happenings. I call them Ghost Stories.

While still working my career job, I worked with an engineer, call him Mike, who got liver disease and died. That was in So Cal at Pt. Mugu… Well, later on my wife and I decided to change things up a little so I quit my job and we moved up north to Southern Oregon to build some houses. My wife at the time, # 4, was a general contractor and we had three other builds under our belts. One day while I was standing behind the dump truck we bought,

I felt a presence and knew it was Mike. I didn't see him physically but there was some sort of vision I had that resembled his figure. It was probably in my mind. But I knew it was him. We chatted for a few minutes. He said he was okay, then it was over and never happened again.

Another story involves a particular house in Ontario, CA. It belonged to a friend of mine. I stayed there several times while visiting from Camarillo where I lived at the time. During the night there seemed to be some force that would cruise thru the house on certain occasions. As I recall it was something like a cold breeze or some feeling that is hard to describe. I remember seeing something like a lite shimmering on an object on a shelf. But don't know what it was. And when I got up to go down the hall to the bathroom, there was a cold breeze-like feeling down the back of my neck. It didn't scare me because I wasn't afraid. I didn't feel threatened. I later determined that it was a friendly spirit of an Indian that had died on the property eons ago. (I have no papers to prove that.)

I was there another night in Ontario with a friend from San Dimas when this phenomenon again appeared and the usual happened. Well, the next morning my friend said "What the heck was happening last night?" So, we both experienced that feeling.

This was shortly before my third wife and I were heading to Washington DC for a new engineering job I had taken. And during that trip I felt the Ontario presence with me during the trip and for several days after we arrived, then it disappeared and I never felt it again.

There are times when I sense that someone or something has touched my leg or thumped me lightly on the head. I feel my dad near me sometimes. Same for my mom. But they were a very strong presence in our lives and they are never out of my mind/head so I might just be imagining these feelings.

Anything else you should know about me? I was introduced to sailing by my father, as were my siblings. We entered several of the New Port Beach to Ensenada races which was quite an adventure. I had a sail boat of my own at one point and sailed the open ocean, exploring the islands of the Southern California coast. During the summer months I back packed into the High Sierras to fish the high-country lakes with my two fishing buddies. I really love the High Sierras. Later on, I built three houses with my third wife. Two in SoCal and one in Oregon.

That experience allowed me to rehab the Colorado cabin into a real home. I sold it for a tidy sum. And, I like Jazz. Especially the Blues. With jazz you either like it or you don't. There's no "Well, it's OK but…" You either get it or you don't. I remember one day in high school, when I was a sophomore, I was used to listening to R&B and one of my buddies said, "How can you listen to that junk. Come home with me after school and I'll show you what great music is."

So, we went to his house after school and he played an album of Dave Brubeck, piano, and Paul Desmond, soprano sax. That was it. It instantly changed my view on music. And from that moment on I was a jazz fan. My favorite artist is Miles Davis, trumpet. I consider him to have been a genius. He never stopped growing in expanding his musical expressions. I have a large collection jazz recordings and play them often.

I enjoy research. Finding out what plants will grow well in the desert where I live and what care they need. I enjoy researching just about anything. Learning new stuff is fun.

Another thing I should mention relates to a spider I saw inside the trash can in my garage. It spun a web right in the middle of the opening. I thought to myself that wasn't a very good place to locate a web. As time went on, I would toss items into the trash can, causing the spider and web to disappear. And each time I did that, the spider and her web would reappear. My thoughts about that were that little spider has a real desire to continue with her pursuit of life. And that thought resonated with me very strongly. That's how I feel about life and living.

19

8-11-54

How do I feel emotionally? I'm very emotionally stable. I feel like I've been through enough years of contemplation, therapy, prayer, collaboration, consultation, vexation, and elation to have a pretty good grasp on how this is supposed to go and how it will end. I almost died when I was 40, and since that time I have cherished being alive each and every day. As the saying goes, "Every day may not be good but there is good in every day." Amen to that!

And physically? Hm. While I'm grateful to be able to do most everything, I've had some physical situations that have altered my lifestyle a bit. I don't think I could ski anymore, and racquetball is out of the question, so there's that. But pickleball is still an option, and chasing the grandkids keeps me young. Sometimes I wonder if I will make it to my Dad's ripe old age of 94 and still be able to swim 600 yards like he did. Some days I already feel 100. Other days, I'm raring to go.

I'm very settled with myself. I try to live my Christian faith (not the thing those Trumpers call Christianity, cause that ain't it by a long shot) and follow the teachings of Jesus. The real Jesus. I just hope he's okay with me swearing, 'cause I've been dropping the F bomb a lot since 2016. But I keep trying.

By all measures, I think I'm in great shape, considering. Turns out there are a lot of body parts you can live without, quite successfully! I have no spleen, no gall bladder, and about 1/3 of my pancreas due to a tumor that was just waiting to take my life. My mom and cousins died of pancreatic cancer, so the hereditary factor was strong. I thank God for my surgeon, Charles Yeo, who saved my life.

Because I have not much pancreas, I am diabetic. And not Type 1 or Type 2, it's technically Type 3C, just to really complicate things! My endocrinologist lists me as a Type 1 because, of course, insurance does not acknowledge 3C. Only 5% of diabetics are Type 1. So, there it is.

But I will say that being diabetic has made my diet a LOT healthier. I decided that I would follow strict protocols for the condition, as I am very attached to my eyes and toes and don't want to lose any of them. Honestly, there's never been a better time to be a diabetic. While I can't do anything to get rid of it, like a Type 2 can, at least they've made it very manageable.

I can walk, run, hike, bike, swim, squat, dance… pretty much everything!

I was rear-ended by a TEXTER in 2019 who didn't even put on his brakes before he rammed me. My car was totaled and I ended up with a concussion, TBI, hearing loss, retinal fold and neck issues, but I went to physical therapy and everything but the hearing has improved.

I was very happily sexually active until my partner passed away last winter (ironically from pancreatic cancer). I have been heartbroken and miss our intimacy very much. But sex for me is more about the person than the act. Especially in my old age. Attraction takes time for me. I am not sure I'm interested in that kind of investment at the moment.

No canes or walkers yet. I am blessed with genes that seem to be very strong and healthy. My mom passed away at 84. At 29, three days after giving birth to me she was diagnosed with bulbar polio, which was years before the vaccine came out. She had many brushes with death, but made it that long. We lost my dad last winter, but he lived (with lots of help from his two daughters but relatively independently) for two years after having a stroke, heart attack, and multiple myeloma. He was amazing, and even at 94, a vital, fun, brilliant human being. BUT if I have to use a cane or walker, I'll be okay with it.

Regarding family, my ex-husband and I are amicably living apart, although we see each other often. We were high school sweethearts that broke up and then got back together seven years later and stayed married for 20 years. I read somewhere that 20 years constitutes a successful marriage, so hypothetically you could have three successful marriages in your lifetime, right?

We have two amazing adult children. One daughter, one son. They both have partners and we love them too. My son and his wife blessed us with two grandbabies who are the loves of our lives. My daughter is a career girl but thinking maybe she and her female partner will have kids one day. I told her that if she wants to have them while I'm still spry it would be a big plus. We love her partner, and they would be amazing parents.

I live alone in the house the kids grew up in. I've been here for 37 years now. I love my home. I told the kids they can just chop me up and bury me in the backyard when I die because I'm not moving. (But I would move if they all wanted to—we're a tribe, a herd.) They both live 23 minutes away from me, but in opposite directions!

COVID wasn't too terrible for us in the sense that we all committed to being together which meant that we had to agree on levels of exposure. We all still wear masks, get our groceries delivered, don't socialize except with one another. It's a mom's dream. My daughter has had to go back into the office, but she's wearing a mask. My granddaughter started preschool, so we're expecting a lot of germs to come our way. But it's important for her to socialize. She's a total COVID baby. Very strange world for her.

My favorite job was being a mom. I was teaching and took leave of absence that turned into forever. I was able to start a consulting company with five other people at that time and that gave me the flexibility I needed so I could raise the kids. It worked out well.

Besides my favorite job, I had a LOT of jobs. I was very good with finance but truly hated it except for being a teller and training tellers. I loved being a bank teller but, besides being a mom, my favorite profession was teaching. Loved, loved. Still in touch with many students, believe it or not.

I do want to be sure this little tidbit is on the books, so to speak:

I started working for a bank when I was 17 (I had to get bonded). I loved being a teller, and I must have been good at it because the bank asked me to train head tellers at their HQ and help them write a policy manual for all of their branches. I was working and going to college to get an education degree. I loved working for the bank. I loved my co-workers and my boss, and what I was doing. I proposed a marketing strategy for them that they gave me a cash award for and used for years.

When it came time for me to graduate, the bank asked me stay on. I thought about it, and then told my boss that I would stay if I could be in marketing and I wanted to make xx dollars. I will never forget my boss, who really liked me, saying, "We don't have females in marketing. We just don't hire women to do marketing!" I said oh okay and turned in my resignation.

The bank called me back a few weeks later, saying they'd changed their mind and I could have the job. But by that time, I was working as a mortgage loan processor so I told them it was too late.

My last job was starting a standards program, and I loved that too! It was a bit hard being a woman in the business I was in, but the esoteric nature of standards opened up a community of like-minded people and lots of nerds from some very cool industries besides the one I was in. I loved my volunteers so much! The association I worked for was wonderful until a new CEO took over. But standards work at least made me feel like the time was well spent. I made exactly half the salary of my male predecessor, by the way!!!

Was the work I did worthwhile? Teaching was worthwhile. I've taught from 3–83-year-olds. I love it. And I've already said my best job was being a mom.

I am not one of those people whose self-worth is wrapped up in what they did at any given time. I have never been bored and always look forward. So, everything in its time. On to the next adventure.

And I am still working! I am a writer. I still write ghost articles for my old industry. I also edit for a big social media company, very part-time, as a subcontractor. It's perfect.

I have a list of things I want to do that is as long as my arm. I'm deeply committed to helping wildlife by creating sustainable habitats. I love trees. So, I have stuff to do. My daughter and I are working on a children's book about saving the animals. 😊

I hope I was good at whatever I did. I think I was? I know I was an excellent teacher, because the school secretary told me so. And sooo many of my students found me on Facebook. I put 150% of myself into a job, and I love people, so I think I was good enough…

Did I make enough money? I was a teacher. I was in it for the glory AND the money.

My ex and I never fought about money. We both had the same philosophy: *Money is a great servant and a bad master*. We didn't have much money, so it's a good thing we didn't care.

My husband was a drummer and I was a stay-at-home ex teacher. I owned a company with 5 other people for 15 years that was very successful (government subcontractor) but we didn't save much $$. So, my last 15 years of working when I went back into bizworld was my chance to build a nest egg.

We had ZERO money when the kids were growing up but honestly, until my ex's drinking got out of control and we drifted very far apart, we lived blissfully simple lives. The kids didn't know how much money we didn't really have. We lived below our means and I probably wore the same sweater for church directory pictures for 15 years, lol. We were raised by depression parents, learned to be frugal and repurpose, make do, conserve. It was fine. We also invested in the stock market and that really paid off. And we bought our house the month before we married. We bought used cars, we made do.

So, had we stayed together, we'd be super-fine. But, I'm fine with what I've saved and have put off collecting social security. Our amazing kids are both very well compensated for their jobs (that they love, which is the driver) so I don't feel pressure to leave them anything. I'd say we're lucky, but we worked at being "lucky."

And we had that white privilege going for us.

It is a little daunting when you age and realize that your wage-earning days are at an end. All my life my mantra has been, "It's just money." You can always get more money (meaning work hard, two jobs if necessary, find a way…don't let money rule you…). Now "getting more money" isn't as easy as it once was!

Do I believe? I don't know where I'd be without my faith. Thanks, God!

My childhood was pretty scarring, although my family probably looked quite perfect from the outside. Too long of a story and boring but suffice it to say that I worked through all of it and from an early age, God and my violin were my solace. I believe in God, in whatever form s/he takes. I believe in the God that is love. I believe in Jesus and have found his example to be the most compelling driver for my behavior; as a leader, as a parent, as a friend…it is so sad to me that people use the Bible to rationalize hatred, bigotry, and murder. So NOT what Jesus said.

I also believe that there is a mind/body connection. Nothing works in isolation—everything is related in some way.

Oh, I totally believe there is life after death, and I've asked loved ones who are dying to give me a sign to let me know that all is well. Boy, you should try that!! It's crazy what's happened in each and every instance. Violin music under my window from my deceased grandmother. A distinctive one-of-a-kind butterfly following me around from my father. And there have been four more.

So yes, there is another act. This is the warmup. I am not exactly sure what heaven is, and I really hope I get the chance to ask some questions when I get there, cause I have a list! But I also think that when we get to heaven, all is revealed. So, our loved ones know everything that is in our hearts, and they stay connected to us.

I said I'm a Christian, but I've never totalllly taken the Bible word for word. There's some disagreement about interpretations of many passages that people cling to when they want to justify some bad behavior. While I love certain books, I focused pretty exclusively on the teachings of Jesus, which are so amazing. However, as I age, I really do find some truths that keep popping up. One is in Ecclesiastes: There is nothing new under the sun. It's so true. There really isn't anything new. The more things change, the more they stay the same. I'm surprised by how far man, as a species, has not evolved!! But I'll keep focusing on the bright spots and praying for world peace. I wish for the world a place that is kind, where all people are respected and loved. Love is everything. All people want to be loved. It's that simple.

What else should you know about me for the book we're all going to write?

I like being old—it takes all the pressure off!! I take every day as it comes, count my many, many blessings, and try to enjoy every sandwich.

Music has enriched my life beyond measure. I think music is spiritual.

I'm a little suspicious of people that don't like dogs, to be honest.

I think that brush with death at 40 gave me some insights that may come later (or earlier) for many people. It certainly had a profound effect on me.

Thank you for inviting me to write all this down!!

20

9-15-48

How am I feeling emotionally? I frequently realize how quickly "time" has flown by. They (Olders) always told me that as the years go by and the older I become, the faster time seems to zoom by. They were/are so right on!

But I feel that I am in pretty good physical shape for my age. And I'm grateful for that.

I'm thinking sometimes that I should get more involved in being part of something bigger, something that is part of the "solution" in making the world a better place. On another level, I feel that creating things from found objects that bring a smile to others is rewarding.

The bounty and beauty of nature means the world to me. I feel so fortunate to have the mountains and ocean just minutes away, where my mind is embraced with happiness while the thoughts of our planet's increasing struggles are temporarily jettisoned light years away. The eastern Sierra's, in particular, have been a heartbeat for me since I was a young child,…finding the trails least travelled for hiking, backpacking, fishing,…always an exhilarating experience. Love the beauty of the rugged peaks, the wind singing amongst the pines, the pristine high-altitude lakes. Nothing more beautiful!

While I feel pretty good about my present physical condition, I must admit that there are now some little aches and pains which I haven't previously had to deal with that are popping up much to my chagrin. I have taken up Pickleball in the past year and a half and feel absolutely synced with this physical activity that now calls to me five times a week. I feel that as long as I can enjoy this game and get that nice exercise with like-minded people, I'm going to keep my youthfulness for many years to come. Just *forget* about age!

Obviously, no cane nor walker for me so far!

About my family, I have two older sisters whom I love equally. One lives six hours north of me and the other lives twelve minutes away with whom I visit once or twice a week. I chose to marry two years after returning from Viet Nam. I was only twenty-two at the time but I really needed a partner for "grounding" after my stint with the service. We stayed together for eight years until our paths parted. We remain friends to this day.

I chose not to have children as my belief then, as it still is, that overpopulation is the overriding problem of the world. Every human being is one more strain on the earth's ability to provide the food, energy, and resources demanded by an individual. I am presently in my twelfth year of my second marriage.

As she previously had two children with her former husband, children hasn't been an issue. We mutually share the love of nature and have had many, many adventures in our numerous travels.

We have different activities as well, which allow for that all important "space" which is vital in a relationship and also allows time for reflection. Our earlier years together had the magic and physical drive that we've all enjoyed as youngsters and which was obviously part of our attraction to one another. That sexual intimacy we've enjoyed has recently transformed into, interestingly enough, a closer, deeper appreciation for each other that is more lasting and sustaining than that testosterone driven obsession of pure sex. Partners for life.

My father was a letterpress printer and as a preteen, I made a buck here and there, sweeping the floors and oiling the presses. And, as time passed, dad taught me the California Job case, and I began setting type for the upcoming printing jobs. Soon I was running the Heidelberg platen press, the folding machines, and the Minabinder, a soft-back book binding machine. I made decent money, and more importantly, I loved the work I had learned to master, especially the printing. Anyway, to make a long story short, my father became a book publisher and some of the equipment I was running became archaic and I eventually said "Goodbye" to all of that and began a new life.

"Where does our food come from?" I wanted to work outside and with those who provide those all-important food stuffs that show up on the kitchen table. I met up with an organic grower who was farming on a beautiful piece of property in the foothills and he offered me a part time job of helping him increase his productivity. Working with him, with the earth, and the end result of taking the cared for produce to the local farmers' markets and interacting with likeminded people was an amazing change for me. Living simply and living happily.

My farmer friend and mentor made a decision with his wife and moved back to Missouri where his extended family resided and began a small farm there. Before his departure, he introduced me to another well-established local organic farmer with whom I became friends. I ended up working with him for about eleven years helping out on the farm, selling at the many farmer's markets, and taking care of his numerous restaurant accounts.

Lastly, I integrated into a management position with the six local farmers' markets for 13 years where I enjoyed my engagement there with *all* those wonderful hard-working farmers who make this whole food thing work. And *all* the wonderful and grateful patrons who regularly come and support the markets.

Today, in retirement, I continue to sell a few canopies and an occasional scale to the growers who need them, but mostly, I enjoy making bird houses and mobiles from beach glass and other found objects. And playing Pickleball!

While I am not religious, I believe in a divine spirit which for me is *nature*. It's so sad that religion seems to be what wars are mostly fought about. Unfortunately, it has and probably always will be… the line in the sand.

21

8-17-36

(I'm not into stories about myself therefore print whatever you want.)

As far as emotionally goes. I am fine. I still know I'm me.

Physically, I can say I'm grateful to be alive because 11 years ago I had liver cancer and part of my liver was removed. They said I had five years to live. Yippy, now it's 11. Wow, I'm still alive. I keep going day by day.

My man partner with whom I live is several (27) years my junior. We have sexual activity occasionally and we are always very affectionate. He is wonderful to me and takes good care of me.

I use no cane nor walker. Until age 75 I played tennis and gym sports, racket ball. Then cancer hit me. I had no chemo nor radiation so, I'm in good shape considering. I do lots of yard work and am concerned about the draught and water problems. But that is good physical exercise. I'm the neighborhood watch so careful on watering days.

About my family. At age 16 a big blow, I lost my mother who was 41. The real challenge was that my father remarried a woman who had a son. For me this was a disaster because she despised me. One day I came home from school and she had given the Salvation Army both my two high school award sweaters, my Bear Cat and my PALS sweaters which meant so much to me and they were never to be seen again.

I buried my most recent husband seven years ago and I was married to my first husband for 23 years. We raised three lovely daughters. In turn I have 10 grand ones and now 18 great grand ones. After my first husband passed, I married another man who had a grandson whom we raised together. That grandson is now successful in business and has two more teenagers who call me Grammie.

My children are pleased with themselves and never caused any heartbreak with jail or crimes. One is 35 now and plays golf daily. For five years he has been voted the best all-around golfer in California by Titlist. They are all happy with their careers. We have a lawyer in Auburn and a police officer in Sacramento. My daughter has worked for 20 years with doctors styling wigs for women who suffered hair loss due to cancer. She lives in VA and sent me every color and cut, snappy wigs when my cancer happened, but I never lost my hair.

My life has had challenges. My work has been rewarding. Worked for 3M a few years. Had 12 employees when I had my marketing company. I worked for a large company as receptionist and operations manager in Pomona. That was fun.

I was president of volunteers at a local hospital for seven years.

All my work was rewarding and fun as I think about it.

We owned a chalet in Lake Tahoe near the ski lift and went there for rest and recuperation when self-employed when we were free to spend time away.

Financially I always made/had enough money and we're doing okay now.

As far as faith is concerned, the Bible is my powerful tool. I have enjoyed teaching Sunday School at several different churches and always loved that.

Also, on Sundays I teach at the old folks' retirement center. That is also a delight for me.

I've had the experience of attending several of my high school friends' funerals. I feel good about honoring them.

And I say again, I keep going day by day.

22

12-21-48

Having many emotions is a slightly stirred and partially blended concept for me. Sometimes I feel as though I have only one emotion. One leveled emotion that holds me on a steady course while other emotions swirl within it like the contrasting batters of a marbled cake. I'm not even sure what it is: that single emotion, but it's able to manifest itself on the surface of me at the appropriate times to conjure the proper responses to the situations in which I find myself. I'm not sure if I feel them. Are my emotions inherently shallow or has some event or series of events built a barrier so great that emotions are not allowed below a certain depth lest they throw that balance off and allow my universe to spin out of control?

In general, I feel extremely lucky and I do feel loved. But I feel inadequate. Disconnected. Unfulfilled. Unfinished. Uninteresting and boring to people yet helpful when they need it. Sometimes I'm too self-absorbed and controlling. Guilty on many levels.

Physically, I've been very lucky. I am very healthy. I look a little younger than my age-number (whatever that means). I don't have any bad joints or pain issues. My blood pressure is good, and I take only one prescription drug, a statin, to keep my lipids in check. I have one issue, an abdominal aortic aneurysm, which is monitored annually via ultrasound to make sure it doesn't grow to the point of rupturing and bleeding out: otherwise, I'm good.

I am still perfectly capable of being sexually active, but with the global pandemic of COVID happening for two and a half years and having no significant other, I have chosen to not have sex with another "in person" for over three years. There is one person I would consider, thousands of miles away, so: occasional "virtual" sex with that person and I would say frequent "in-person" sex with myself are the extents of my sex-life these days.

No cane or walker. I'm totally mobile and independent, still drive and travel alone whenever I get the opportunity.

I'm proud to have five living and loving siblings, four brothers and one sister among whom I am second to the oldest. I also have one grown loving daughter and two wonderful grandsons both in university. They live in Texas, and now, after living in California their entire lives, I live in Baja California, Mexico so we don't see each other as often as I would like. I recently moved into a house where I could live alone with an ocean view. It's more expensive to live alone but the freedom to practice and play the piano, or, have rehearsals with singers without worry of disturbing a housemate is priceless.

My day job was a union job doing ticketing for live events: concerts and Broadway shows. I was a member of IATSE Local 857: Treasurers and Ticket Sellers. Before that I was a musician and a member of the Musicians Union: pianist, accompanist, musical director, and composer/songwriter. I continued part time with my music while the ticketing career basically took over as the main source of income.

I feel good with that decision as it allowed me to retire with decent social security and a union pension monthly and I'm now free to pursue music again without depending on it for income. I think my work was worthwhile. I do not miss the ticketing work, but I have really missed playing the piano and I was actually very good at both jobs.

There were times when I did not make as much money as I would have liked, but there were also times when I made more than enough money. Currently, financial considerations are not an issue. I have enough and I have what I need.

Regarding spirituality, I am a recovering Southern Baptist. I've always considered myself spiritual, but I do not believe in a "sky-god" nor the hypocritical dogma and trappings of organized religion or the HATE. If I believe in a god from whose likeness we are created I would look to the universe. We ARE made of the same components and I believe life after death is that our energy does not die but returns whence it came: unconsciously into the universe.

What else should you know about me? Even though I was married to a woman and have a grown child and two grandchildren, I have always known that I was sexually attracted to the male gender. I had many romantic and sexual affairs with women, but my preference is and has always been men. When I was in college and fell in love in another male student for the first time, I realized then what that meant and finally realized what it was.

I was engaged to a woman at the time and felt that it was dishonest and unfair not to tell her, so I did. It was 1968 and she wasn't prepared to accept that information so we broke up. After that, though, I told every woman I thought I might become involved with that I also had affairs with men, so I was not one of those who hid it from their girlfriends/wives. It didn't seem to bother them, until I got married to a woman that I had been having an affair with and lived with for several years.

During the course of that relationship, I met a young man I fell in love with, and we found a place to live together, which we did for a year. He became so abusive I left him and eventually the woman with whom I'd broken up with for him and I got back together, finally married and had a child. We were divorced when my daughter was six. My ex-wife and I made sure I kept my relationship with my daughter. When I was in my 30s, I decided I was going strictly with my first preference and dated only men after that.

23

3-24-44

At this stage of my life I'm experiencing something I never expected. My mother, who is 105, is living with me as I am her full-time care giver, she has dementia. I'll come back to that later.

I'm in good health for my age. I don't take any prescribed medications and only vitamin D3 for my bones.

I was married and have two wonderful children and two granddaughters. My oldest granddaughter is studying to become a doctor, very proud of her. My youngest is still in grade school and at this juncture of her young life she wants to be a teacher. My son lives 3 hours away and I don't get to see him very often. My daughter only lives 20 minutes from me so I am able to see her and my youngest granddaughter more often.

After graduating from High School I went to Junior College for 1 semester then enrolled in Beauty School. I worked as a beautician for several years and really enjoyed it until I developed an allergy to the hair care products. I was under a Dermatologist care for 6 months and couldn't get my hands wet. It was a difficult time for me. After that I wasn't able to go back to hairdressing, sad for me because I loved it.

Good thing I had taken accounting classes in High School so I went on to work in an office atmosphere. I enjoyed that and was good at it. I'm happy I had something to fall back on.

I was a stay-at-home mother, that was very important to me as my mother had to work. Walking home from school every day, all my friends went home to their mothers and I went home to an empty house. I wanted to be home for them. I wanted to see their smiley faces and their art work etc. I didn't want to miss out on that. I had to return to work when they were teenagers and I don't think that was a really good time for me to do that but I had no choice.

Back to taking care of a loved one who has Dementia or Alzheimers, it is the most difficult job one could ever have. It gets more difficult as they descend deeper into it. You will need more patience than you could ever imagine. She also has Macular Degeneration and doesn't see very well so she is unable to read anymore and has a hard time seeing the TV and my large clock.

I have to help her dress and undress, put her hearing aids in and taking them out, and her shower. She needs a walker as she is very unstable on her feet. Her walker is a regular walker not the one with a seat.

It starts out very slowly, usually with the memory loss of a word or words, which we don't think much of in the beginning. We all go thru that, it's normal. Then they don't remember where they put things or where things belong, for example putting something in the fridge when it doesn't belong there. Soon they don't understand simple concepts, are unable to take medications correctly and don't remember what they're for, the list goes on and on.

Any change in routine or another place, as in a 2 day get away, is very confusing for them and they can become very anxious or frustrated.

Many changes occur as they progress on this journey and it's different for each person. You can't give them choices as it's too confusing and difficult for them.

My mother is in a delusional state, she's always asking me where did those ladies go that were here, or where her mother went because she was here earlier, when is my mother coming to pick me up, doesn't she live with us etc. You have to learn how to play the game and give them an answer that will satisfy them for the moment. The first time she asked me where her mother was I told her she had passed away several years ago, well that didn't compute. I had to learn how to come up with something quickly to satisfy her. I realized she was living in the past. That's where some go as sometimes those memories are still there. So now I answer in the present and that seems to satisfy her.

She has had, for a very long time now, a habit that drives me nuts and that is she picks her teeth all day and spits all over. She always thinks food is stuck in her teeth and she will choke and die if she swallows it. She has it in her head that you aren't supposed to swallow your saliva.

They lose everything, I call it the 4 C's, Confusion, Cognition, Comprehension and Concentration. They are very good at masking it at first, but the longer you talk to them you will realize something isn't right. They talk in what I call The Loop. It seems to go well until you realize they are saying the same thing again and again.

These are only a couple of examples of how it is. There are many more. It is very challenging, frustrating, up-setting and sad to see it happening and you can't do anything about it.

It's so difficult finding time for oneself just to do the simple everyday things in life. I have to be with her, and I mean right in her sight, at all times. I have to tell her when I leave the room for a moment, because if I don't she thinks she's alone and gets scared. Even if I tell her, she forgets.

I joined a support group for people who take care of a loved one who has Alzheimers or Dementia. We meet once a month for 2 hours. Our facilitator gives each one of us a chance to discuss what has transpired since our last meeting. It has helped me tremendously to be with others who are experiencing the same thing. We also learn from one another and bounce ideas off one another. Only those who are going thru the same thing or who have already gone thru it really know what it's like. No one can really imagine what it's like unless you live it 24/7-365, to understand the trials and tribulations it presents. It's nice knowing you're not alone. If someone is experiencing something they know nothing about, such as Sundowners, our facilitator will get someone to come in to tell us about it.

I would consider myself more spiritual than religious, in that I don't belong to or go to church regularly. I believe we should treat everyone the way we would like to be treated and to be kind to every living creature on earth. We should try to love and respect each other. I believe what goes around will come around. Having a positive attitude also helps, try to always see good over evil.

24

10-1-46

I was born in the Fall of 1946. I'll soon have my 76th birthday.

For the most part I would judge myself as doing well, perhaps very well. My day-to-day emotional state seems steady and certainly reasonably happy. Physically, I am also able to take care of my personal needs, help around the house and yard, fix meals, drive whenever and wherever I might want to go. Driving would include 2 or 3 trips per year in the hundreds of miles and navigating congested urban highway systems. I am cautious, but not daunted by occasional encounters with heavy and treacherous urban traffic.

My self-image is positive. I find purpose and value in what I do, though it is often repetitive and mundane. I feel I am benefiting myself and serving my family and friends by being a bit proactive in reaching out, making visits, engaging in minor projects and keeping family and friendship ties intact. I have served the larger community as a volunteer on boards or foundations and in service clubs, but, honestly, I've little interest in resuming those activities. I feel more fulfilled in keeping in touch and engaging with my children, relatives and friends.

I am private and prudish enough to refrain from detail on my sex life, but I will say that I am occasionally active.

My physical condition is good, not great, but I do not use a cane or a walker. I have a chronic arthritic condition, but with modest use of over-the-counter anti-inflammatory medication there are very few days I have any sense of activity-limiting pain. I do have some sense that I have a bit of balance impairment and I am careful in the bathroom and shower. I don't turn or get up too quickly and have had a couple episodes of my leg falling asleep while sitting too long in one position. Fortunately, I've not fallen in such circumstance, but I've felt I've come close a time or two. That said I am careful and believe I am able to take on more tasks than many others my age might try.

My family consists of my wife, my first wife died many years ago, two sisters, two children, three grandchildren. I live with my wife, my sisters, children and cousins live in other communities or states. Most live within a couple hours of us. We live in a single-family home in a nice community and nice neighborhood. We employ a lawn service company, but spend some time tweaking the yard as needed. We do not have cleaning or other in-home help.

Before retiring I was in the business world and part owner of a small service-oriented company. I found my work essentially enjoyable and fulfilling. Earlier in my life I had enrolled in a couple post college educational programs to increase my professional development. Eventually, and with some degree of being in the "right place at the right time," I was reasonably successful at what I did.

I enjoyed working with my partners and company staff. I feel strongly that I was a team player. I did not gauge success as a personal accomplishment, rather a group effort. I felt pride in our company's philosophy of seeking good people, providing above peer average compensation and good health and retirement benefits.

My post college professional development gave me the confidence that I was knowledgeable in my field and I was able to work with larger and more complex client circumstances than many of my peers. That, and a good opportunity led to my realizing some financial success. I would say that I did make "enough" money.

I have never been a spendthrift. I did have a time in my career that was rough financially and I never wanted to re-visit the anxiety that can create. Our business and family spending habits were not lavish, we worked and lived comfortably, needed nothing we could not afford and limited our wants. We were prudent and savers. That and good fortune allowed me to retire from the working world at a relatively young age. I'll have to say that the balance I've achieved in my life is satisfying. I did enjoy my work life and the people I worked with… but I do not miss the daily routine of working.

Current financial considerations are not troubling. I feel I should be okay through the remainder of my life. My home is owned with no mortgage, I have adequate funds to pay my bills on a timely basis, we currently have no family health related financial concerns. I do grouse a bit about the fluctuation in the stock and bond markets, but I am not obsessed about it. Sure, I would love to have a greater net worth, but I don't feel it would improve my quality of life or have much affect on how I spend my time. If anything, greater wealth would probably be shared within our family or philanthropic causes I support.

I am a practicing Christian. I am less involved in church activity than earlier in my life. I attend church regularly, averaging a couple times per month. I no longer serve on church boards and on Sundays I do not attend in person I sometimes tune in for worship via the internet. It is hard for me to imagine life after death, but that is a matter of faith. I also have the notion that in a way we live on after our passing at least in the memories of those who knew us. When those people pass on our existence fades into the pages of eternity…

My last thoughts on being an "older" center around memories of those who have gone before me. Though I consider myself in the younger or middle ranks of older, I am sometimes staggered by the passing of the many people who have been factors in my life. Many were friends, too many were family. I was actually present first at the death of our infant daughter, then some years later the death of my mother, then years after that the death of my first wife and the mother of my children, finally at the death of my father. I have been right there as last breaths were taken, I witnessed deterioration and life ebbing away before the last moments. My mother's last hours were gruesome to witness. My father's death was the only one that came suddenly and he is the only one of these who died older than I am now.

When my wife was in cancer treatment, there were many friends who professed their support and with whom I felt comfortable talking about her illness. She lived a few years after diagnosis and most of that time enjoyed a good quality of life. Ironically, at one time I counted a half dozen friends who had shared their concerns about my wife, who had been in apparently good health, and then died before she did. We were not "old" people. Everyone I'm remembering was in their 60's.

These last 20 years or so have simply underscored the non-permanence of our existence, the threads by which we cling to life. I do not dwell on these losses. Frankly, I probably live my life without thinking much about my own death. But the memories are reminders and each year there are more familiar names that disappear from the roles of the living. Right now, if I think of my four closest friends, one died in January at 75. Another has three diagnosed issues of medical concern. Another is suffering from the ravages of chemotherapy and stage 4 cancer. The fourth had cancer treatment starting about fifteen years ago and receives ongoing treatment every couple months. I too am among the ranks of those who deal with one kind of cancer or another. I am doing well. I am checked every three months or so. I have good and accessible care.

I am thankful for the life, family and friends I've had. Those of us who are still here agree we've had good lives. We would like some more time and have never thought being here is anything short of a miracle.

25

8-21-43

I am emotionally sound. Always a glass half full type person.

I take great pleasure in my five grandchildren and one great grandchild. I was 19 when I married and proceeded to have four children by the time I was 25. So, I guess you could say I grew up with them. I have to laugh when people complain about raising one.

I only wish I lived alone. My adult daughter and her husband are currently living with me due to hard times that befell them four years ago. I'm working on getting them to move along. I want my privacy back!

Physically, I'm in pretty good shape. Don't use a cane or walker. Do everything myself. I drive myself. I'll go anywhere, just point me in the right direction.

Not overweight. I eat healthy. Like to cook and bake. A lot of recipes from my mother and grandmother.

Not sexually active at the present. Not from lack of interest but from lack of a partner.

My sisters and I are very close. One lives in Phoenix and one in Switzerland. A brother in Georgia. So, I have a few really nice places to visit. And have been to all.

This is pretty funny, I do some caregiving for my daughter's mother-in-law who is 85 with dementia.

For 20 years I worked for friends of mine who had a hospital pharmacy inventory business. It involved a lot of travel which I loved. And yes, I was good at it. After that, I worked for a Dodge dealership as a biller for 15 years. If I do say so myself, I was very good at that job. That was a crazy time. A lot of male admirers. Trouble was, some of them were married. I forgot to mention, I was divorced by then. I made enough money.

I'm very comfortable with most of the tech stuff. I worked on computers my whole adult life. I text, FaceTime, google and use my iPad for everything.

I was raised Catholic. So yes, I have religious beliefs and know in my heart there is an afterlife. As a matter of fact, I visited my mom and dad's grave today to say a prayer and put a holiday decoration on it. Both my mother and father have visited me. My mother passed 10 years ago and we can still smell her scent in one of my bedrooms. Very comforting.

If you need any more detailed answers. E mail me.

26

2-19-47

How do I feel? That is so hard to answer as it changes daily for me. I prefer to be home alone a good deal of the time. I relish the night/days that my husband is out…which are many. I find being with groups of people to be exhausting and I want to go home earlier than my husband. I prefer to have conversations with one person at a time. I am annoyed by boring people or people who interrupt others.

The biggest change for me occurred when I retired. That's when I became less social. I was very social when I was working. Going out to lunch, meeting up with small groups and lots of meetings. But I'm much less social now. Which is fine until I begin to feel left out. I want to be alone until I've been alone for too long. Then I want to find someone to be with.

My husband is even more social than when we were working. He has something going nearly every day or night of the week. Sometimes I feel guilty about not having enough to do. Am I lazy or antisocial? I watch a lot of television. When he is home, he plays games on his computer while he "sort of" watches TV.

Lately I've been convincing myself that my level of activity is fine, acceptable, and will do. I was at a reunion recently where someone asked me what I do with myself. I answered "nothing." I think I felt ok with that. Physically I have little energy, have lots of headaches and stomach issues. I have medication for the headaches that help sometimes and not others. My stomach issues are acid indigestion, nausea, and can result from the headache meds. I get both headaches and stomach aches from food i.e. sugar, alcohol, tomato sauce, red meat and spicy food. Both of these "aches" have been going on for a long, long time.

I have also been on antidepressants since my father died in 1993. I had been seeing a therapist before that. I stopped seeing a therapist probably 25 years ago. I couldn't find anyone in my town that was satisfactory. I'm still on antidepressants. Two meds for stomach, four for headaches including an injectable, two meds for blood pressure, one for herpes, and one for preventing the return of breast cancer. I had breast cancer, stage 2b, in 2013 and 14. I came through breast cancer fine.

We are sexually inactive. Maybe three or four times a year. Some of this is because my husband had prostate cancer that severely diminished his ability to get an erection. It is also because my desire has diminished which happened after my hysterectomy. In addition, my lack of desire was there from the beginning of our marriage. This was problematic then but no longer is.

I don't use a cane or a walker.

We do not have children and it's just the two of us living here. We married in our early 40s and tried for a couple of years to get pregnant. Didn't happen.

I was promoted to Division Manager for Public Health in Health Care Services in the two years before I retired. Before that I worked as Administrator for the AIDS Program for about 22 years. I was good at what I did and received information that others felt that way also. I miss the work and coworker interaction but I was glad to retire when I did. The work was worthwhile but just as I left the AIDS Program the state removed all funding from the program. It felt as though much of the work we/I did was just eliminated. I did make enough money that allowed me to travel and save enough for retirement.

Financial issues are not a consideration for us. We both have pensions, money we saved and funds we received from the death of my mother. We are currently remodeling our kitchen which is very expensive but we can afford it.

I do not believe in life after death. I have no religious or spiritual beliefs.

I think that is it for me.

27

11-7-44

How do I feel? Emotionally I feel great and good physically. I am a walker and a gardener and very social. I like to keep moving and need projects to make me happy.

I am in good physical shape. I do sometimes have asthma and I am very proactive with taking meds to keep me from having flare-ups.

My husband passed nine years ago and I don't want to be a nurse or a purse.

I use neither a cane nor a walker.

I have two children and four grandchildren.

I live by myself with my dog and I like it that way.

Before retiring I was controller for a corporation. It was worthwhile but I don't miss it because

I volunteer. I was good at what I did and I made enough money. And now I still have enough money. Seven years ago I became a practicing Catholic. I was brought up an atheist. I have peace and I do believe.

What else should you know about me? I am a very positive person and I enjoy helping the "elderly" and love working in my garden where I harvest the veggies and bring them to elders who cannot work in the garden anymore. I am very fortunate because my daughter helps me in the garden.

I also have most of my family near me and I enjoy the mixed ages not just people of age. Engaging with the youth is key for me in that they have so much ambition, fun, and I can learn so much from them. I didn't want to text and several years ago my kids told me that that's' the only way they will communicate with me…lucky me I embraced the "new" and I am not left in the dark.

I am proficient using my computer since the 1970's and can use many applications and last year I learned how to use a database for fundraising. To me learning is the best gift I can give myself.

I do not look at the news or watch much TV and I am selective with social media. I tend to back away from people who are negative, and if I need to engage, I put mental Teflon around myself so that the negative vibes won't penetrate.

Lastly, I enjoy having a dog who is a young Lab, she keeps me company and on my toes. I just enjoy the simple things in life; family, friends, flowers, the sun, moon, stars, sky, trees, birds, bees, butterflies, and children playing together on our street. My journey is what I make of it and not to put off today to what can be done tomorrow.

Passed down from my grandmother's eulogy…

My Credo is…*it's not how long you live but how you live!*

28

5-7-45

I feel great. I live in an ocean of love.

Though my body is now quite old and afflicted in the many ways old bodies are, my life has never been better. My knees and hips whine a bit (my left knee is just begging for surgery I'm prepared for, but in no hurry). My heart has misbehaved, I passed out at 60mph sixteen months ago when my pulse dropped to a leisurely 20bpm. It was a very brief nap of, perhaps two seconds, and I got out of the oncoming lane without overcorrecting into a ditch, a good outcome, no?

Meds and a pacemaker seem to be doing the trick. As old men do, I've had prostate cancer, or it had me. Either way I won with help from science. Had a bit of a problem with stricture secondary to irradiation of the offending organ, but that's been sorted as well.

No, I don't use a cane or a walker, but while I think my balance is typically good, it's not what it was.

Am I sexually active? Somewhat.

We have, I believe, an absolutely beautiful marriage. We have occasional abrasive moments, but they are minor and quickly resolved. We have tender concern, pleasure in each other's company and pastimes we enjoy together, all suffused with an easy intimacy.

We have no children, but love the children of our extended family and of our many friends, and are loved by them.

After HS I joined the navy to get away from my family. Post navy I worked at a variety of trades, carpentry, telecom, custom photo printing, light industry.

My first marriage was ill-chosen, not that I was in the least prepared for a well-chosen one. In the summer of 1969 as a consequence of a suicidal gesture by my wife I entered psychotherapy. I always describe it as the world went from black and white to color. I left my wife and became determined to work in the field of counseling and therapy.

To that end I started college at 26, whilst also continuing treatment to become sufficiently mature for the work I was determined to do.

Was my career worthwhile? Very much so I believe, working to support folks struggling with social and/or psychiatric problems. Loved the work.

Was I good at it? For some folks, I was excellent, for some, utterly useless. I did my best. I've said that for a third I was definitely good, a third I probably didn't do much for and a third not sure. I loved the work. After I retired, I volunteered for eight years at a local non-profit. Again, I loved my work. But I don't miss it, I have a large number of close friends, so I have plenty of opportunities to "be there" for someone. I sure don't miss committees and meetings. Anyway, I'm too busy now, I don't have 40 hours to spare every week.

We have all the money we'll ever need. We saved assiduously and my wife inherited an equal amount or more. Till I was in my 40s I rarely had more than $20 left on payday. Now I can give generously to forty different causes and buy anything I want, short of a Lamborghini. No worries.

I've long enjoyed the art of carpentry and enjoyed creating a few beautiful objects. In recent years I've taken up silk painting/dyeing. It has given me enormous joy. And as the silk I'm working with is hemmed scarves, it is a joy I'm able to share. Art is boon for the spirit, create it if you dare, have it in your life at a minimum. And Music.

I've done a fair number of drugs. I've been a regular marijuana user since 1963. While I was working, I used pot two or three evenings a week, now I like a little edible most evenings. I like marijuana, but the drug that had the most impact on my life has been LSD. In my youth I tried a number of drugs. Snorted heroin twice, fabulous, but not worth wrecking your life for. My only significant addiction has been tobacco, I shook it, with help. But LSD deeply changed my perspective on being human, our relationships, our psyches and our flaws. It changed my thoughts and feelings regarding the unanswerable questions, death, infinity, god, love.

For many years I liked to say I was raised not to believe in any religion with more than one member, having been raised by a virulently anti-Catholic Irish Catholic father and a secular Russian Jewish mother.

The older I've gotten the greater I find my love for humanity has become. That feeling of oceanic love that one feels on the drug ecstasy has taken root in me. My experience has been that it is a short step from loving humanity to imagining an ocean of soul connecting all living creatures in the whatever the universe is.

I can imagine what soul I possess returning to the ocean, but self ends, I imagine.

I love to imagine, but I don't imagine an afterlife and I don't need to.

Life has been and continues to be, Grand.

One of my favorite stories took place on a crisp autumn night around 1950. I should have been home as it was already dark, but I stood in the street looking up at the clear night sky ablaze with stars and knowing I was standing on a rock hanging in space. I knew that it was awesome and incredible that we existed at all. I also knew that the adults around me seemed to have forgotten or never seen. I promised myself that I would try to remember. I did lose track for some years, but that little boy's awe has never left me.

29

9-25-23

Good morning!!!! I would be happy to contribute to your book but I don't really understand how I do this. I could answer all the questions and as my son said, I could write some silly poetry; please give me some more information on how I should do this? Example; question, "How do I feel about growing older?" Answer; "It's hard to describe; part of me says "Whoopie, I'm almost 100!!!" Another part of me says, "Wait a minute; do you really want to do that? Just think how much trouble you might be to your dear loving sons."

    I feel a little confused about all these questions; physically I feel fortunate for surviving cancer and polio and still enjoying pretty good health.

Not having a living husband, I am not sexually active.

I sometimes use a cane but always a walker. It's my companion and I dare not try to walk without it.

Family; you'd better believe it! Two sons, four grandkids.

I live in Wesley Manor.

I was an elementary school teacher and then a secretary. I definitely felt it was worthwhile and I do miss working. You ask if I was good at what I did; I have always been told that I was but who knows?

Teacher's salaries were considered very generous and I certainly felt well paid. As far as I know, financial considerations are not an issue. To my knowledge I have enough money; my son is my financial advisor and he says I have enough money to last my lifetime. I have no idea of what range I would consider necessary.

I definitely believe in a life after death and think, as the song says, "We will understand it better after a while when all the saints of God are gathered home…" I don't consider myself a saint but I do believe we will all be gathered home!!!!

I think maybe I told you about the poem I wrote? Well, here it is.

A sample of my poetry:

> "Did you ever feel like you don't know why,
> you look up in the sky but you don't know why?
> Why am I still here and not up there?
> You bow your head and say a prayer.
> You know God loves us and we love Him too!
> Without His love, what would we do?
> So, let's trust in Him; He knows what's best.
> Let's just close our eyes and get some rest!!
> Tomorrow is another day,
> a day to work, a day to play.
> Whatever is to be will be, that's what I've heard!!!
> I may be singing like a bird!!!
> Amazing Grace, how sweet the sound!!!!!"

My identity? 9-25-23. Thank you and good luck with your book!!!!!

30

And So

The people who willingly participated and even enjoyed participating in this project were from all over the United States and one from Canada. And what have we learned from these wonderful Olders that we did not know or understand before? A few things and several that they had in common. Since I know many of these people personally, as I read their stories, I wanted to jump on the phone and talk to them about some of these things. Mostly things I had in common or problems for which I had solutions. I am by nature an empathetic person; it was easy for me to relate to most of what I read. I'm thinking the readers will feel the same way about many of these stories.

This is not a scientific research project, so I don't think we can generalize from all of these except for a few things.

I thought that we could learn more from people who were infirm in one way or another. The more infirm people did not have the energy or interest to participate. I also found that some of the people whom I know best felt the questions were too personal and were too shy to write about their private lives and feelings for me to read: my brother, one of my best friends, and my immediate neighbors.

As I said in the beginning, people do things in their own time, and some of the people who had agreed to participate needed prompting and prodding to get something to me. It was all fine. As I have said previously, just like 20- or 50-year-olds, olders do things at their own pace in their way and in their own time.

Two people gave me their stories handwritten. One of those does not own a computer. Living these days without a computer cannot be easy. Another did not feel comfortable enough writing on the computer and dictated his story to a mutual friend.

I regret now that I did not ask more about technology. We were all born long before there were such things as computers, and we had to learn about them and how to use somewhere in our 40s. My grandsons sat at and used their own computers at age two. So we are of a different generation. Some of the stories offered information about their technical skills, and that was interesting. A couple of people said they were very comfortable with this tech age and used the computer for everything. The 99-year-old was back and forth with me on email several times.

And a few more mentioned how difficult this age is because of what customer service has become. It is almost impossible to speak to a human. One is required to fill out this and click on that and do this that and the other thing often just to get a simple question answered. And horrors if you happen to click on one wrong number or letter. You are lost. For the youngers, it is an easier matter. For us olders, it is frustrating and difficult and usually takes up a lot of time.

I also did not ask about driving. I believe all of these people who contributed or at least most of them are still behind the wheel, doing their own shopping, etc. We all see older drivers, especially women, cruising the highway at below the speed limit. It's okay. We have rights too.

So what did they have in common? All had aches and pains from mild to somewhat degenerating. All talked about parts wearing out and things not working as well as they used to. Several talked about increased visits to doctors and how tiresome that is. All felt it was necessary to be active to try to keep things working.

Several mentioned the sense of loss, as I did. Friends pass away or move away to be with their children. And our own children move away. There is an acute sense of loss when these things happen, and at our age, they happen all too frequently.

Several said they now found politics and sometimes politics coupled with religion troublesome in this country. Also, how religion was too closely mixed with business. No one mentioned any names or what exactly bothered them, but they felt the country was on a wrong track. Certainly no one likes the violence that is evident because that is plain scary. As I write this, a critical election is taking place. Perhaps their concern was related to this election.

I think people are curious about sexual activity among the olders. Our stories lead us to believe that about one-third of these people still have occasional or regular sex with their partners. Most said sexual activity was a thing of the past; but if they had a partner, regular playfulness, dancing around, patting, and petting were frequent and enjoyable. In other words, affection between partners is common. Some of the single people were not interested in having a regular girl or boyfriend and preferred being on their own.

Many said they felt younger inside, that is, not in their bodies but in their thoughts and feelings. Younger than they really were in age. An interesting idea…feeling younger while your joints hurt, you've increased doctor visits, and your balance seems to be leaving you.

To all, family meant a lot. A few lived alone, by choice, and liked it that way. At the same time, they talked lovingly and appreciatively about their families. Only one who participated lived in an adult care facility, so we didn't learn much about that large set of people.

Some women said that the most important thing they did in their lives was having and caring for their children. Their wonderful grown children gave them great joy.

All felt that the work they had done in the past was worthwhile and that they did that work well. Most did not miss working, some because of now doing regular volunteer work. Several missed the camaraderie of the workplace, a team of people working together to accomplish a shared goal.

The issue of having a religious or spiritual belief system was very interesting. It seemed that a strong religious connection gave people a strong sense of security, well-being, and happiness. There was a difference between the Christian sort of believing and the more intellectually considered spiritual kind of believing, guardian angels, and that sort of thing. A couple went to great lengths to explain their beliefs. And to some, nature itself was their God and their grace and their true caring. Very interesting. There are some good lessons here from people from both persuasions.

Several people had experiences with, we'll call them visits from, deceased loved ones or others. One called them Ghost Stories. They are described in separate people's stories, and I have requested people to share if they had such experiences. There were also several people who did not believe in an afterlife nor in any kind of higher being. They didn't appear to suffer from this lack. And one who said he did not believe in an afterlife mentioned having feelings of the presence of deceased former wives.

Hmmm. It is clear that to ever have such experiences, one must be open to them.

One of the issues I thought would be discussed the most was hardly mentioned, that of the isolation experienced by many Olders. I'm thinking that since these people were all pretty well, they were out and about, not so much experiencing that isolation.

In my own piece here, I mentioned how I believed the Asians and others had it right. The family lived together with the old folks sharing the living arrangement and being part of the activities of the family well into old age. Such a nice idea.

In this country, the children of Olders may live many, many miles away from their parents, making visits difficult, if not impossible. All the people I know love to have a visit or a call from one of their children. It just makes them happy. I also think that the isolation is experienced more by the Olders who are homebound and infirm, and of that group we had few participants.

Checking out the world life expectancy charts, the United States is way down, but most have women living longer than men and living into their mid to late 80s. To what do we attribute these people in our group having these long lives? Genetics?

Physical activity? Good diets? I guess we don't really know, do we? Maybe it's pure luck.

And thank you to all who contributed these lovely stories. None were offered that were rejected, so we were fortunate in how very good they were. A couple of them were experienced writers. And interestingly, about four were in some way involved in performance—theatre, acting, musicianship, directing, whatever.

Again, thank you to all for sharing your interesting life experiences. They made engaging and thought-provoking reading. And many thanks to my husband, Norman Russell for the help in reading, editing, ideas, and general support he gave to this effort.

ABOUT THE AUTHOR

The primary author, Janet Benner, PhD, at age 86, is herself an Older. She had been looking for a way to assist older people in her neighborhood, some caring for infirm spouses and some infirm themselves. She started a group for 80-something women that inspired her to believe a book would be the best way to reach lots of older people and those who care for them. She has authored three other nonfiction books: "*Parent Survival Training*," "*Football: Mysteries Revealed for the Feminine Fan*," and "*Smoking Cigarettes: The Unfiltered Truth*."